Naturally Healthy
MEXICAN
COOKING

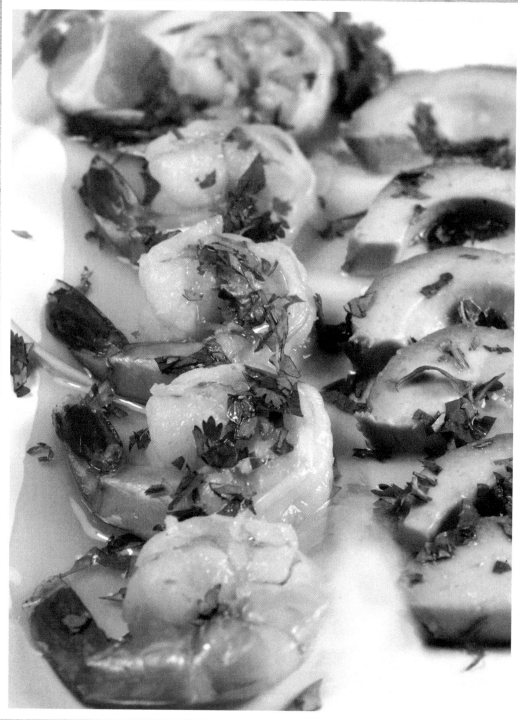

Aguachile-Style Ceviche

Naturally Healthy

MEXICAN COOKING

Authentic Recipes for Dieters, Diabetics & All Food Lovers

JIM PEYTON

UNIVERSITY OF TEXAS PRESS, AUSTIN

Joe R. and Teresa Lozano Long Series in
Latin American and Latino Art and Culture

Requests for permission to reproduce material
from this work should be sent to:
    Permissions
    University of Texas Press
    P.O. Box 7819
    Austin, TX 78713–7819
    http://utpress.utexas.edu/index.php/rp-form

The paper used in this book meets the minimum
requirements of ANSI/NISO Z39.48–1992 (R1997)
(Permanence of Paper). ∞

Design by Lindsay Starr

LIBRARY OF CONGRESS CATALOGING-IN-PUBLICATION DATA

Peyton, James W.
    Naturally healthy Mexican cooking : authentic recipes for
dieters, diabetics, and all food lovers / by Jim Peyton.
        pages cm
    Includes bibliographical references and index.
    ISBN 978-0-292-74549-0 (pbk. : alk. paper)
    1. Diabetes—Diet therapy—Recipes. 2. Low-calorie diet—Recipes.
    3. Reducing diets—Recipes. 4. Mexican cooking. I. Title.
        RC662.P49 2014
        641.5'6314—dc23
                                                    2014018327

doi:10.7560/745490

Contents

Preface

I USED TO STRUGGLE with keeping my weight and cholesterol in check, especially when I indulged my passion for Mexican food—until I learned how to do it with no loss of pleasure and satisfaction! The first step in solving the problem was to understand why I enjoyed food so much. I realized that a good meal, besides the obvious answer of great taste, has the power to banish stress to a distant memory and that I unconsciously relied on that. Since then I have discovered that countless others use food as a way to deal with the pressures of daily life. I also learned that many will not give up their favorite foods, even after dire warnings from their physicians.

It followed that, for food lovers, the key to dieting and eating healthily could have nothing to do with blanket approaches to things like fat and carbohydrates, and certainly nothing to do with eating food they disliked. The more logical road to health through diet would be to eat meals with good nutrition profiles—not too many calories or too much fat, sugar, and unpronounceable chemicals—but that food must be so delicious that it provides the all-important reward. Only then would we welcome it as a permanent part of our lifestyle as opposed to a barely tolerated diet to be abandoned at the first sign of success.

I soon discovered another important truth: it doesn't matter how healthy your food is if you eat too much of it. Fortunately, foods that are nutritious, delicious, *and* made with high-quality ingredients are so satisfying that most people are content with smaller portions. The simple and rewarding approach I envisioned and now use can be summed up as *eating food that is delicious and healthy in moderate portions.*

At first I wondered if it would work with Mexican food. Were there enough healthy and truly delicious recipes—recipes good enough to be served in restaurants—that didn't take all day to prepare? It did work, even better than I thought possible. I quickly discovered that there are more delectable, easy-to-prepare Mexican dishes with exceptional nutrition profiles than I imagined when I began this exploration over forty years ago. This book contains the commonsense advice and outstanding recipes that have been successful for me, and there is no reason they cannot work for everyone who loves good food!

Acknowledgments

TO ALL THOSE WHO provided advice and help, including Bill Lende, Candace Andrews, Elena Hannan, Lucinda Hutson, Elizabeth Johnson, Lewis and Mary Fisher, Dr. Donald and Judy Gordon, Dr. Jerald Winakur, Linda Thoennes Farr, Diana Barrios, Angela Shelf Medearis, and, above all, my ever-supportive wife, Andrea. I also want to thank the too-numerous-to-mention cooks who, over so many years, have chronicled Mexico's cuisine, providing invaluable reference material for those who follow them. Finally, I want to thank the professionals at UT Press who did such an amazing job of turning my scribbles into something to be proud of, most especially Casey Kittrell, Leslie Tingle, and Kathy Bork.

Naturally Healthy
MEXICAN COOKING

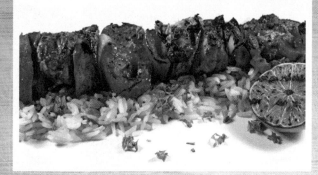
Swordfish Shish Kebab

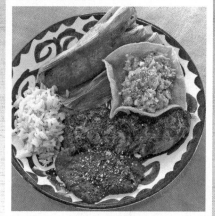
Steak Combination Plate

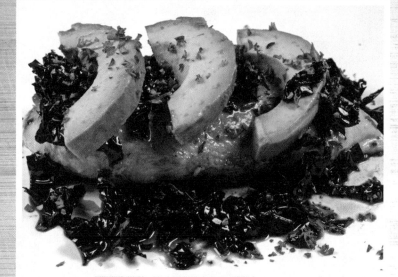
Pollo Agridulce

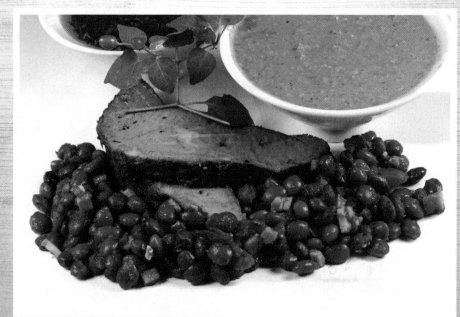

Potato Gorditas

Santa Maria–style Tri-tip Steak with Pinquito Beans

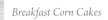
Breakfast Corn Cakes

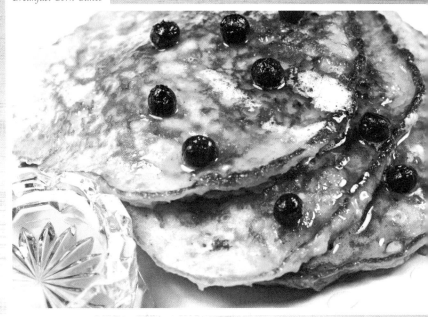

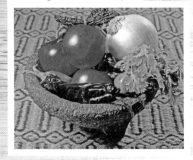
Salsa Ingredients in Molcajete

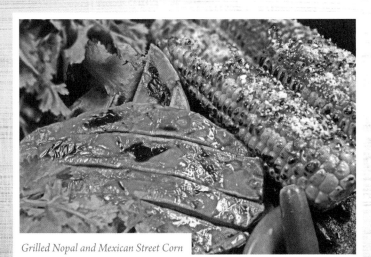
Grilled Nopal and Mexican Street Corn

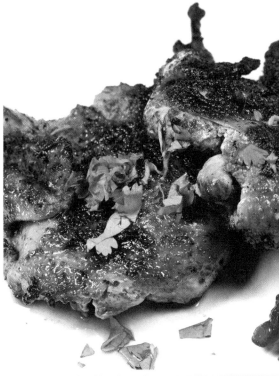
Grilled Quail

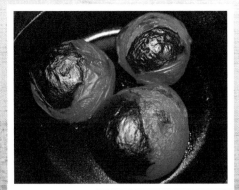
Roasted Tomatoes

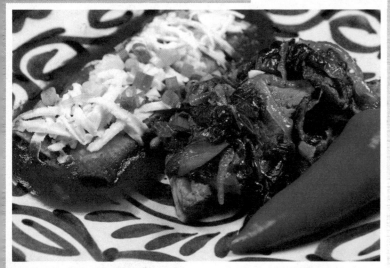

Steak Served with Enchiladas

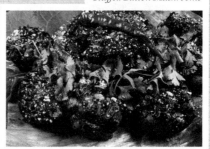

Stuffed Button Mushrooms

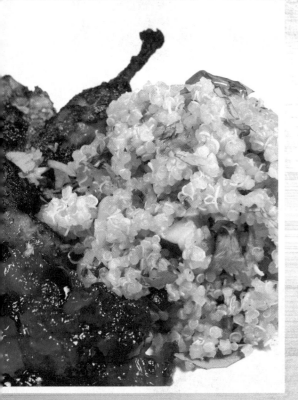

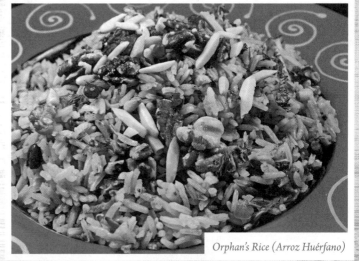

Orphan's Rice (Arroz Huérfano)

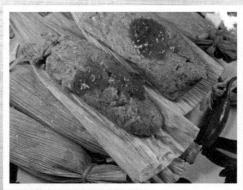

Fresh Corn Tamales

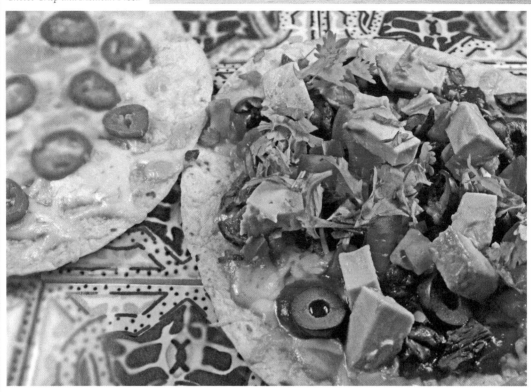

Cheese Crisp and Mexican Pizza

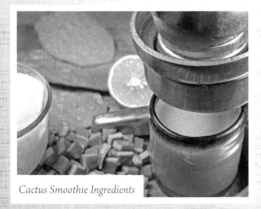

Cactus Smoothie Ingredients

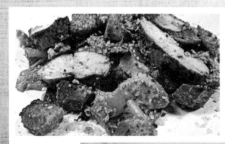

Caesar Salad

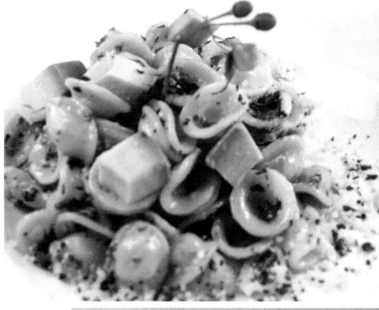

Pasta Arriera

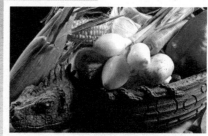
Assortment of Vegetables

Shrimp Adobo with Grilled Squash and Mexican Street Corn
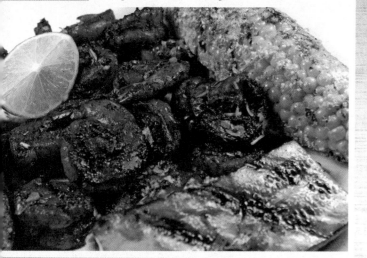

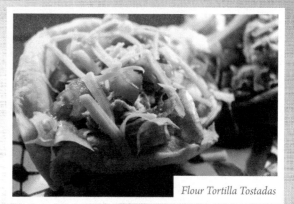
Flour Tortilla Tostadas

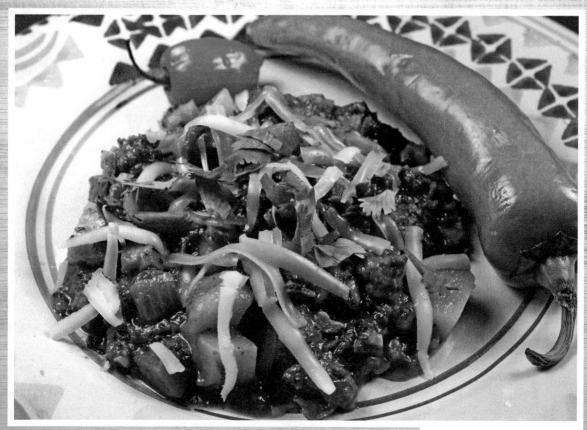
New Mexico–style Green Chile Stew

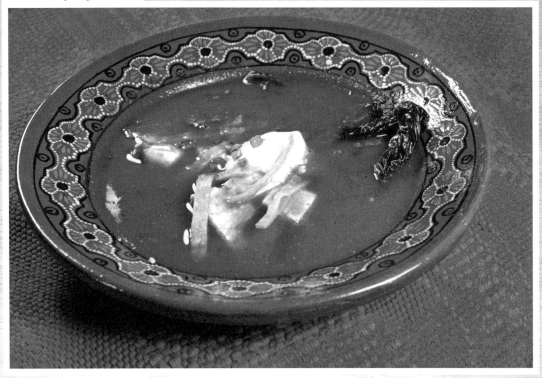

Tarascan Soup (Sopa Tarasca)

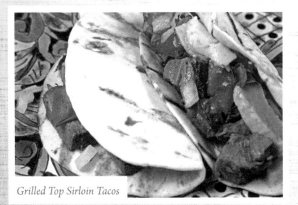

Grilled Top Sirloin Tacos

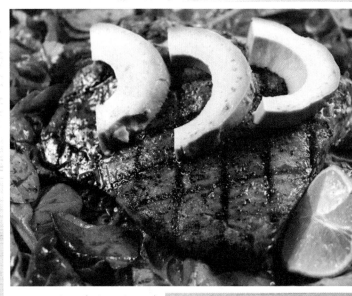

Coconut Salmon (Salmón de Coco)

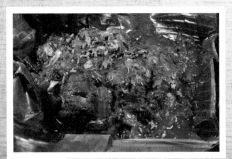

Pollo Pibil

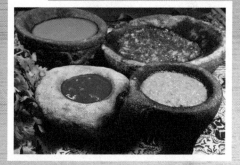

Salsas

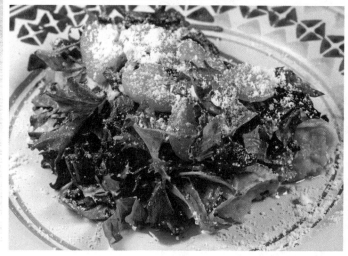

Sweet Potato Enchiladas

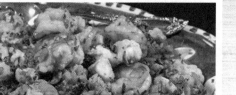

Arroz a la Tumbada

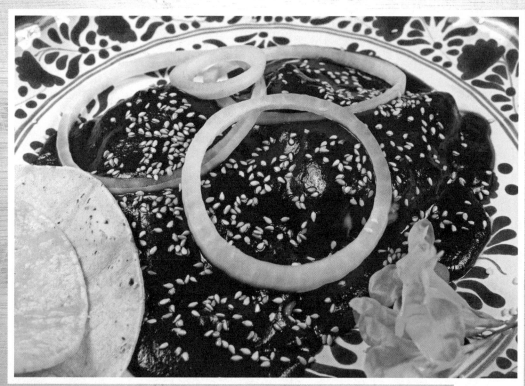

Mole Sencillo

INTRODUCTION

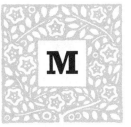

M Y LOVE OF MEXICAN FOOD began with my first bite as a kid. I sampled it initially in San Diego, then on trips to Baja California, Arizona, and New Mexico, and later in Texas, where I attended college and graduate school. By the time I finished my education, our southern neighbor's cuisine had become a significant part of *my* culture.

I had not cooked much Mexican food because my favorite dishes were readily available in restaurants where I lived. In 1970, I moved to Hawaii and discovered that, at the time, the fiftieth state had no decent Mexican restaurants. Fortunately, my wife shared my passion, and we spent vacations during the next few years in Mexico and the U.S. Southwest, collecting recipes and then experimenting in our kitchen. That process accelerated after we moved to Scottsdale, Arizona, and resulted in my first book (see the bibliography).

My interest in Mexican food increased in tandem with my understanding of the subject and its history, and I wrote three more cookbooks. I also gained an appreciation for the benefits of a healthy diet. Fortunately, I discovered that there were so many delicious Mexican recipes with wholesome nutrition profiles that there was no reason to make substitutions that altered what made them appealing in the first place. By contrast, while they are certainly good for you, many of the recipes advocated by diet books and nutritionists fall well short of what appeals to people who take delight in good food. For these people, each meal should be a celebration of life, and there are an abundance of nutritious Mexican dishes that achieve that goal. If that objective is not met, most food lovers will quickly revert to their favorite comfort foods.

There can be much more to diet than just dropping a few pounds. For some people it is a matter of life and death. Mexicans and Mexican Americans suffer inordinately from diabetes, especially Type 2 diabetes, which can sometimes be controlled by diet. Putting that together with the fact that, after a lifetime of study, I have learned a fair amount about Mexican food, I decided to work on a cookbook for diabetics. I was surprised to learn that what diabetics are supposed to eat is almost identical to what everyone should eat: a well-balanced diet that is reasonably low in calories and fat. The primary difference is that diabetics must be able to precisely control their intake of carbohydrates. With that knowledge, I decided to broaden the project from a focus on diabetes to what you will find in this book: a collection of delicious and healthy recipes from all aspects of Mexican cooking that are made with natural ingredients and authentic recipes.

Diet and Healthy Eating

The purpose of this book is to provide tasty recipes with good nutrition profiles for lovers of Mexican food. As summarized in the preface and expanded below, that goal is the result of the most important lesson I have learned during a lifetime of trying diets designed for everything from losing weight to lowering cholesterol. The secret to any such regimen is to enjoy the process so much that you do not think of it as a diet but as a part of your lifestyle that gives you pleasure. Because many, if not most of us, unconsciously use food as a reward for dealing with the stress and other unpleasant things that occur daily, diets often fail because so many "diet" foods do not supply that necessary reward, and people refuse to eat them.

So how do healthy foods become a bona fide daily reward? Some Hollywood stars have private chefs who specialize in "spa" food. They prepare dishes that have the proper nutrition profile and are so tasty that even the most demanding gourmets look forward to them. Others have their food sent to them by diet services that have learned to prepare low-calorie dishes that people enjoy. Most of us, however, do not have the money for a full-time chef or the time to prepare complicated dishes ourselves, nor is it realistic for most people to have their meals delivered to them for the rest of their lives.

The solution is to identify dishes you really enjoy that are low in calories, fat, carbohydrates, and any other personal considerations. They should also be affordable, nutritious, and reasonably easy to prepare. You don't have to crave them with the same passion as your most beloved comfort foods, but they must be good enough so that instead of feeling deprived between splurges, you look forward to each meal and are content with the reward it provides. The recipes in this book are designed to help you do just that. Food should make you happy, you should look forward to each meal, and you should enjoy eating the kinds and amounts of it that allow you to meet your goals.

How much we eat can be even more important than what we eat. So in addition to reducing the frequency with which they eat high-calorie foods, many people must also reduce their portion sizes. Just as they will change what they eat if they enjoy it enough, people will also reduce their portions if their meals are well prepared, made from quality ingredients, and otherwise satisfying. How important this can be and how it works is made plain by an examination of what has been called the French paradox. Research indicates that the French have just over one-third the deaths from heart disease that we do in the United States, second only to Japan. Where the paradox arises is that studies indicate that the French consume more saturated fat than Americans, and while the French have about the same rates of high blood pressure and HDL (good) cholesterol as we do, their total levels

IT'S THE CALORIES!

Even though the science of nutrition is constantly changing, with once-forbidden foods such as eggs and coconut oil recently being given the seal of approval, virtually all nutrition experts agree that we should eat a well-balanced diet of vegetables, fruits, whole grains, lean meats, poultry, and fish. That diet will work every time for most people—as long as it contains the proper amount of calories and, for diabetics, the right balance of carbohydrates, fat, and protein.

Regarding the issue of calories, carbohydrates, and fat in diet, a study published in the February 26, 2009, issue of the *New England Journal of Medicine* (Sacks et al. 2009) followed people whose diets involved different amounts of those items. The only constant was that they all reduced their calorie intake by 750 per day. After six months, each group averaged nearly the same weight loss: thirteen pounds. After two years, each group had kept off an average of nine pounds. The conclusion was that it was the number of calories—regardless of where they came from—that was the key to weight loss.

of serum cholesterol are higher and their heart disease and cancer rates are much lower (Fraser 2000).

Nutrition experts believe that smaller portions and several other factors contribute to the lower disease and obesity rates in France, in spite of the fact that the French consume more saturated fat and have higher cholesterol readings—the very things that we have been told are killing us. Some of those healthy practices include the following:

- ▶ The French eat much smaller portions than Americans—from 30 percent to 70 percent less. This means that even if they are eating fatty or other high-calorie foods, total calories consumed may be considerably lower than in this country.
- ▶ The French consume an average of 60 percent of their daily calories by 2:00 pm versus only 40 percent in the United States. That means they get their calories when they need them, for energy during the workday, rather than just before they go to sleep.
- ▶ The French eat more slowly than Americans. Studies show that from the time we begin to eat, it takes fifteen to twenty minutes before the brain sends a signal to reduce our appetite. While many Americans complete a large meal in less than that, the French may just be finishing an appetizer, soup, or salad.
- ▶ Because of their love of fine food, the French avoid processed foods. Instead, they use the very finest ingredients they can afford to prepare their meals from scratch, which makes their smaller portions better and therefore more satisfying.
- ▶ The French do not obsess about calories, carbs, sugar, salt, and fat the way Americans do. They simply eat delicious foods made with high-quality ingredients in relatively small portions and regard their meals as an important and enjoyable part of their life and culture.

Diabetes and Diet

Most people diet either to lose weight or to become healthier and more energetic. Unfortunately, increasing numbers are forced to change their eating habits because they have diabetes.

There is no special diet for diabetics other than the same healthy regimen that is recommended for everyone—a variety of nutritious foods. However, while the diet may be the same in terms of the type of foods consumed, the meal plan for diabetics can be quite different. "Meal Plan" refers to the amounts of specific foods, such as carbohydrates, fats, and proteins, that are eaten at each meal and on a daily basis. Since each person is different, there is no one meal plan that works for everyone. For example, the needs of an overweight individual are different from those of someone

DIET IS A NUMBERS GAME!

One vital item to remember is that eating well is a numbers game, one that can easily work to your benefit. For example, if you eat three times each day and substitute just one healthy meal for one that is less good for you each week, you will have bettered your diet by nearly 5 percent. If you do that for two full days of meals a week, you will have improved your diet by nearly 30 percent. Another example comes from a recent study. In an April 2009 article in *JAMA Pediatrics*, the authors concluded that reducing added sugar in the amount of one soda per day or increasing fiber intake by the equivalent of one cup of beans per day produced improvement in risk factors for Type 2 diabetes (Ventura el al. 2009). Constantly bear in mind just how important even a small change can be to your lifetime average.

who is underweight. Therefore, diabetics should work closely with their physician and a registered dietitian to create the best plan for themselves.

One thing that is increasingly thought to be important for diabetics and everyone else is the type of carbohydrates they consume. Those that cause the body's blood sugar to rise most slowly are preferred. That rate of absorption is listed in what is called the glycemic index. The lower a food is on the index, the more slowly it will raise blood sugar. I had hoped to include the glycemic index for the recipes but found that there is still not enough data in the calculation program. However, lists of ingredients with their glycemic indexes are widely available, and it is a simple matter to avoid high-index items in favor of lower ones.

Mexican Cooking and Nutrition

Before the Spanish conquest, Mexico's Indian tribes had what by today's standards would be considered a nutritionally excellent diet. Their staples were corn, beans, and squash, invigorated by the addition of chiles. They also consumed many other vegetables and a large number of fruits. Their animal protein came mostly from seafood and lean game animals. While they ate the right kinds of food, their main challenge was to get enough of it.

The Spanish brought cows, pigs, chickens, sheep, and goats to Mexico. Those meats and their by-products, such as milk, cheese, eggs, and lard, added a great deal of fat to the Mexican diet. And to protect Spain's domestic growers, the Spanish government made cultivation of olive trees in Mexico illegal, causing people to use lard instead of better-for-you mono-unsaturated olive oil, as they did in Spain.

The Spanish also brought their recipes with them, and the two foodways merged to form a brand-new cuisine. For the most part, the Mexican ingredients and recipes prevailed as Spanish ingredients were incorporated into the Indian recipes for tacos, tamales, stews, and entrées. Corn, beans, other vegetables, and fruits remained atop the resulting food pyramid.

While a few of the new dishes were indeed laced with fat, most of them were well balanced in terms of protein, fat, and carbohydrates. Just as important, most Mexican cooking was developed in rural areas, using high-quality ingredients with no chemical additives and little or no processing. That was true even in some of the cities, such as Puebla, Oaxaca, and Mexico City.

Some of Mexico's most famous dishes, including the *moles*, were developed in urban convents by Spanish nuns working with their Indian servants, using produce grown lovingly in their own orchards and gardens. To this day, Mexican home cooks and chefs take great pride in the quality and nutritional goodness of their ingredients. In fact, much of our organic produce now comes from farms in Baja California originally developed to support the area's burgeoning restaurant industry.

DIABETES

Insulin is a hormone produced by the pancreas that converts sugar into energy. Type 1 diabetes occurs when the pancreas produces no insulin or not enough of it. Therefore, Type 1 diabetics have to take insulin injections. To keep their blood sugar levels as normal as possible, they must also balance their food intake with their insulin intake and expenditure of energy.

Type 2 diabetes used to develop later in life but is now affecting people at younger and younger ages. It accounts for about 90 percent of all cases. It occurs when a person becomes resistant to the effects of insulin or when the body stops producing enough of it. Many Type 2 diabetics are obese, and that is thought to be a principal cause of insulin resistance, so weight loss is a primary goal. A combination of a healthy diet and exercise allows some patients to avoid taking medication.

THE MYSTERY OF CORN

Because of its success as an easy-to-grow staple in Mexico, corn was exported to the far corners of the world—from the United States to Europe to Africa. But a serious problem arose: everywhere outside of Mesoamerica that people adopted corn as their staple, they became ill with a sometimes-fatal disease called pellagra. It was not until 1974 that scientists solved the mystery of why corn was unable to serve as the primary food elsewhere: when the kernels are eaten with their skins intact, the human body is unable to assimilate and process some of the essential nutrients it needs to remain healthy.

What was—and is—different in Mexico is that Mexicans consume corn primarily in the form of tortillas, tamales, and *atoles* (corn-based gruels). Before those items are prepared, the corn is first made into a masa (dough) called *nixtamal* through a process called nixtamalization. That procedure involves cooking the dried corn in an acidic solution of slaked lime (or sometimes ashes or seashells) to soften the corn so that the skins can be removed from the kernels. With the skins gone, humans are able to assimilate the essential nutrients.

Previously, scientists thought that the reason for eliminating the skins was purely culinary—in order to produce a smooth dough. Perhaps the skins *were* originally removed solely for that reason, and the fact that the process allowed humans to use it as a staple was nothing more than a coincidence. If so, it was one of monumental significance.

WHILE AMERICANS ARE FAR MORE knowledgeable and sophisticated about food than they were even a few years ago, some misconceptions nevertheless die hard. Among them is the notion that Mexican food is fattening or not good for you. The main reason for that has to do with our narrow exposure to our southern neighbor's cuisine.

The first large wave of Mexican immigrants to the United States came to escape the devastation of the Mexican Revolution in the early twentieth century. The majority arrived with little or no money and just in time to experience our Great Depression, so large numbers of them were forced to live in poverty. To feed their families, they adapted their recipes to our least expensive ingredients, and necessity often forced them to use large amounts of energy-giving lard. What was missing in the immigrants' diet were the traditional soups, entrées, seafood, fresh vegetables, and fruits that are the mainstay of interior Mexican cooking.

When those Mexican Americans opened restaurants, Anglos found their offerings to be addictively delicious. The downside was that many of the menu items relied on large quantities of cheese, fatty meats, and fried foods. And they often used partially hydrogenated lard instead of the pure lard of Mexico. That is not to say that all Mexican American recipes are unhealthy. Far from it! This book includes many highly nutritious, low-calorie dishes from the various schools of Mexican American cooking in Texas, New Mexico, Arizona, and California. Nevertheless, those early views continue to be perceived as reality, doing Mexican cooking an enormous disservice.

Ingredients

AGAVE NECTAR

In pre-Hispanic Mexico there was no sugar, and one of the only sweeteners came from the agave plant, in the same family from which tequila and mezcal come. The native population tapped the plant in much the same way we tap maple trees to get maple syrup. The resulting sweet liquid was called *aguamiel* (honey water). After it is fermented it becomes pulque, a slightly alcoholic beverage. When the *aguamiel* is heated, the carbohydrates convert to sugars. The reason the product is popular among health enthusiasts and diabetics is because it is much lower on the glycemic index than sugar— under 30 as opposed to over 60. (The higher an item is on the index, the faster it enters the bloodstream and the less desirable it is for diabetics.) Nevertheless, like any natural sweetener (and most other good things), it should be taken in moderation. In fact, many characterize agave nectar as being over-processed (some is and some is not) and containing as much or more fructose as high-fructose corn syrup. It is generally used in this book in very small amounts in place of sugar, honey, or other syrups.

ANNATO SEEDS AND ACHIOTE

The deep reddish seeds of the achiote tree have been used for centuries as colorings and in makeup. Some historians believe they are the original reason for referring to Indians as "redskins." More recently, they have provided the coloring for margarine and yellow cheeses. Cooks in Yucatán state use the seeds as a principal ingredient in their most popular seasoning paste, achiote. Both the seeds and the paste are readily available in Hispanic groceries, although making your own paste with the seeds is usually preferred.

BANANA LEAVES

Banana leaves are used to wrap foods, such as fish and tamales, before they are steamed, baked, or broiled. They impart a unique flavor, and when the steaming packets are opened at the table, they make an effective presentation. Some Hispanic markets carry the leaves fresh, but mostly they come frozen. They must be softened to make them flexible enough to wrap food without splitting. The best way to do this is to run the leaves back and forth over an open flame for a few seconds. To keep from burning yourself, I recommend using a pair of kitchen tongs or the high-temperature professional mitts used to pick up very hot items while grilling. The leaves can also be softened by steaming. They have a shiny and a dull side, and the shiny side should be the one next to the food.

BUTTER SUBSTITUTE

I enjoy butter as much as the next person, but because it is so high in saturated fat, I try to limit its use to splurges. Fortunately, there are a number of butter substitutes that are quite tasty and much lower in calories and saturated fat than butter. Many of them also contain beneficial items, such as omega-3 fatty acids. My favorite butter substitutes to date, based on calories and taste, are the Smart Balance Buttery Spreads. To replace unsalted butter I like the low-sodium one, and instead of salted butter I use the one made with extra-virgin olive oil. Both have only 60 percent of the calories and about 28 percent of the saturated fat in butter.

CHEESE

Cheese was brought to Mexico by the Spanish, and like so many other foods, as soon as it arrived Mexicans began to create their own distinctive versions. A visit to any modern Mexican marketplace will confirm that the result is a dizzying number of Mexican cheeses, especially when they are multiplied by their regional variations. Fortunately for cooks in the United States, there are just a very few types needed to prepare the most popular Mexican dishes, and either they or decent substitutes are readily available in most parts of the country. The following is a short description of each one. A special note to the lactose intolerant: in almost every case you can substitute Spanish Manchego cheese for mozzarella or other melting cheeses, and Pecorino Romano will work to replace *queso cotija*. Although the taste is different, if you like it, goat cheese can be used in place of *queso fresco*.

Fresh Soft Cheeses

These cheeses are difficult to melt and are usually—but not always—used as garnishes for items like tostadas.

Queso fresco. *Queso fresco* is a fresh cheese that is used to garnish everything from *antojitos mexicanos* (literally, little Mexican whims) to soups, but it does not melt well. Probably the best substitutes are Muenster or the soaked feta mentioned below under *queso panela*. Because neither of those is a great stand-in, we are lucky that *queso fresco* is now available in most supermarkets.

Queso panela. This fresh, fairly soft cheese has a distinctive texture that the great Mexican chef Ricardo Muñoz describes as porous and spongy. It is used to garnish *antojitos* and is essential to the famous Tacos Potosinos. Fortunately, good versions are often available in U.S. supermarkets. Feta, which has a similar texture, is often suggested as a substitute, but I find its flavor is usually so much stronger than *panela* that it doesn't work. However, if you start with a very mild feta, break it into small pieces, and soak them in several changes of ice water over about 30 minutes, it will serve in a pinch.

Requesón. *Requesón* is fresh cheese that is similar to ricotta, a mild version of which makes a decent substitute. It is used very much like *queso fresco* to garnish everything from gorditas to enchiladas, but is also used in salads and to stuff peppers.

Semifirm Cheeses

These are the melting cheeses used to make quesadillas, as a topping for enchiladas, and for dishes like *chile con queso* and *queso fundido*.

Queso asadero. This cheese is especially popular in northern Mexico. It is made partially with milk that has been allowed to become slightly sour, giving it a wonderful tart flavor. It is otherwise similar to *queso* Oaxaca. I have never found a good version in the United States, but *queso* Oaxaca or mozzarella make decent substitutes.

Queso Oaxaca or *quesillo*. This delicious cheese is very similar to whole-milk mozzarella and string cheese, which are excellent substitutes. It is perfect for everything from quesadillas to enchiladas.

Hard Cheeses These cheeses have a texture similar to Parmesan and are usually grated and used to garnish anything from hot tortilla chips and tacos to soups, pasta, and egg dishes.

Queso cotija and *queso añejo*. For all practical purposes, these cheeses are identical, although *queso cotija*, whose name comes from the town of Cotija de la Paz in the state of Michoacán, is the most common version in the United States. They are hard like Parmesan and slightly salty. They are sold in small blocks and finely grated, which I think is the best way to buy them. The grated version may not last as long, but what you don't need at the moment can be kept in the freezer. Although some people suggest Parmesan as a substitute, I think its flavor is too distinctive. Fortunately, *cotija* cheese is widely available in the Southwest and frequently in other parts of the country.

CHICKEN BROTH I use either homemade chicken broth or a very good packaged one that is low in sodium—70 milligrams per cup. If you use one with more sodium, be sure to decrease the recipe's salt content accordingly.

CHILES Since pre-Hispanic times, Mexico's most basic food staples—corn, beans, squash, and chiles—have been grown together in small garden plots called *milpas*. Besides the positive nutritional aspects of chiles, which include vitamins C and A, their main purpose is to provide spice to an otherwise bland diet. Following are brief descriptions of the chiles used in this book, all of which are reasonably easy to find.

First, I want to correct one of the greatest misconceptions in the culinary world, one that is often repeated by people who should know better—that a major part of a chile's heat is in its seeds. That misunderstanding arises from the fact that the majority of the heat is actually in the placenta, or veins, of the chile, found next to the seeds.

Many Mexican chiles come both fresh and dried, and often each version has a different name, which can lead to confusion—until you know them well, when the different names actually make the ingredients more readily identifiable.

Fresh Chiles *Poblano*. Probably named for the state of Puebla, poblano chiles are the large, triangle-shaped ones used for stuffing and to make *rajas*, and wherever a mild chile with lots of flavor is desired. Because of their thick skin, they are almost always roasted and peeled before using. Poblanos are often mistakenly referred to as pasilla chiles in California.

Jalapeño. Probably the most common chile found in the United States, jalapeños are named after the city of Jalapa in Veracruz state. They are used widely in salsas and are also often pickled and stuffed. They are very similar in both heat and taste to serrano chiles.

Serrano. About the same length but much thinner than jalapeños, serrano chiles have a similar level of heat and taste, although I prefer them for the hint of citrus in their flavor.

Habanero. Only about 1½ inches in length, these lantern-shaped chiles are usually a beautiful light orange when ripe. They are also the hottest of the traditional Mexican chiles and are most often used in the cooking of Yucatán state.

Anaheim. Sometimes called California chiles, Anaheims are similar in appearance to green New Mexico chiles but are usually milder. Like poblanos, they are often roasted and peeled and used for stuffing and to make *rajas*, especially in California.

Green New Mexico. Although similar in appearance to California's Anaheim, these chiles vary in heat from fairly mild to very hot, depending on the variety. Each of them also has its own sophisticated flavor profile, which, like fine wine, depends on the soil and microclimate where it is grown. The chiles grown around Hatch, New Mexico, are generally considered the best.

Dried Chiles   Specifying the amount of dried chiles for a recipe can be difficult. The larger ones, such as the anchos, New Mexico, guajillo, and pasilla varieties, come in different sizes. We could use weight, but it also varies depending on how dry the chiles are. The best dried chiles still have enough moisture to be quite flexible but, especially in stores with little turnover, they can become brittle, and the difference in weight can be considerable. The recipes are designed for chiles of average size, something that will be quickly learned with a little experience.

Ancho. Ancho chiles are dried poblanos and may be the most popular dried chile on either side of the border. Mild and fruity, they are an important component of most *moles*, are used in many sauces, and are even served stuffed. While not a perfect substitute, in many situations, 1 tablespoon ancho chile powder can be used per chile. As with poblanos, ancho chiles are often called pasillas in California.

Pasilla. The pasilla chile is the dried chile chilaca. They are long, thin, and nearly black. Sometimes referred to as pasilla negra, they, like the ancho, are quite mild and, with their chocolaty flavor, are another staple of *mole* recipes. They are also used in many sauces and salsas.

Chipotle. Chipotle refers to a smoked and dried jalapeño. The drying process shrinks the chile enough so that the heat is concentrated in a much smaller area, making the chipotle much hotter than a jalapeño. They are sold in two forms: dried and canned. In the latter case, they are rehydrated in a catsup-like adobo sauce. For most purposes, the canned version makes an excellent, easy-to-use substitute for the dried ones.

Guajillo. Guajillo chiles resemble dried New Mexico chiles but are smaller. Next to the ancho, they are probably the most popular dried chile in Mexico. They are fairly mild and used in many different sauces and salsas.

New Mexico dried red chiles. These are the dried version of green New Mexico chiles. They have the same sophisticated, earthy flavor and the same range of heat, from mild to very hot. There is no substitute for them in the cooking of New Mexico except that, in many cases, a high-quality pure New Mexico chile powder works well.

California dried red chiles. These are dried Anaheim chiles, which are often used in California and parts of Arizona in the same way that ancho and New Mexico chiles are used in other places.

Chile de árbol. Usually about 1½–3 inches in length and quite slender, these fiery chiles are used primarily to add heat to salsas and sauces.

Chile pequín. These tiny football-shaped chiles are extremely hot and are used in much the same way as the chile de árbol.

Chile Powder

Most commercial chile powders contain other spices, such as cumin and oregano, as well as salt—sometimes a lot of it. They also almost always include ground-up seeds, which make the powder more bitter than necessary. Whenever recipes call for chile powder, that means pure chile powder, usually made from ancho, New Mexico, or pasilla peppers. I usually buy my ancho chile powder from Penzey's Spices and the New Mexico powder from the Santa Fe School of Cooking. My favorite is their Authentic New Mexico Red Chile Powder with medium heat, formerly called Chimayo-style Chile Powder.

CINNAMON

There are two types of cinnamon, and they are quite different. The most common one found in the United States is made from the bark of the cassia tree. It is dark brown and has a strong, spicy-sweet taste. The cinnamon used most often in Mexico, *canela*, is the true, or Ceylon, cinnamon. It is beige to light reddish brown in color, and while it is considered more aromatic than cassia bark cinnamon, its flavor is less spicy and, I believe, more subtle and sophisticated. It is definitely more appropriate for Mexican recipes.

CORN FLOUR

Corn tortillas and tamales are traditionally made with *nixtamal*, which is prepared by boiling and soaking dried field corn with a little slaked lime to rehydrate the kernels and loosen the skins so they can be removed. Once that is done, the corn is ground into a wet dough. To make *nixtamal* more accessible, producers began redrying the processed kernels and grinding them into flour. The main brands are Maseca and Masa Harina. The former makes a fine grind for tortillas and general-purpose use and a coarser grind for tamales. All you need to do is add water and knead the dough. Tortillas made with the old-style *nixtamal* are considered superior because their texture is slightly more elastic. Some cooks at least partially solve this problem by adding about 1 tablespoon all-purpose flour per cup of corn flour.

EPAZOTE Epazote (*Dysphania ambrosioides*, formerly *Chenopodium ambrosioides*) is an herb that is found wild in most parts of the country, but many people are unaware of it. Although its flavor is difficult to describe because it does not really resemble anything else, it is strong and somewhat gaseous in a way that mysteriously enhances the equally distinctive flavors of items like huitlacoche, mushrooms, and black beans. It is used in Mexico with those foods, especially in quesadillas and tamales. If possible, use it fresh, as the dried leaves are bland and tend to fall apart.

HOJA SANTA *Hoja santa*, saint's or holy leaf (*Piper auritum*), is used all over southern Mexico and especially in Oaxaca to flavor everything from stews to soups to tamales. It is sometimes called the root beer plant because of its flavor, which resembles licorice or anise. It is easy to grow from cuttings and makes a lovely addition to any garden or landscape. It dies off during very cold weather but comes back in the spring.

HOMINY In Mexico, stews made with hominy are referred to as pozole, often spelled *posole* in this country, especially in New Mexico. The most popular type of hominy is *cacahuacintle*, a starchy corn that produces large, tender, round kernels. Pozole is almost always made by cooking the dried corn until it is tender, the same as cooking beans.

In this country most of the hominy comes already cooked in cans, and that is a problem for two reasons. First, canned hominy does not have nearly the same fine taste or al dente texture as cooked dried hominy. Fortunately, dried hominy is readily available on the Internet, and I get mine from the Santa Fe School of Cooking (listed on the site as "posole" in the Specialty Foods section). As a lesson regarding food industry economics, bear in mind that it takes only about ⅓ cup of dried corn to make the approximately 1½ cups you get in a 15½-ounce can of hominy.

The other problem with canned hominy is that it contains a lot of salt, usually over 1,500 milligrams in one can. When I make it from dried hominy, I put just ¼ teaspoon salt in the cooking water, in addition to some chopped onion, jalapeño, garlic, and oregano. It takes a good 3 hours to cook, or about 5 hours in a slow cooker, and much of the added salt is discarded. You can tell when it is nearly done, as the kernels will appear about to burst, and their texture will become pleasantly al dente. For the above reasons, all nutrition calculations for hominy are based on our home-cooked recipe, Pozole Side Dish (page 76).

HUITLACOCHE Sometimes spelled *cuitlacoche*, huitlacoche is a black mushroom-like fungus that grows on corn, often taking the place of some of the kernels, and it is considered a delicacy in Mexico. Although it is difficult to find fresh huitlacoche in this country, the Latin food company Goya, which serves nearly all Hispanic groceries and a majority of regular supermarkets, sells a canned version that is very tasty. Just ask your market to order it from them.

JAMAICA *Jamaica* is the dried flowers of the hibiscus plant (*Hibiscus sabdariffa*) or the drink made from them. The flowers are a deep magenta in color, and that is transferred to the tea they are made into. They are readily available in supermarkets in the Southwest and in Hispanic groceries and some health food stores in other places.

LARD Traditionally, lard has been the most important fat in Mexican cooking, ever since the Spanish Crown banned the planting of olive trees to protect domestic growers. It is essential for an authentic taste in things like tamales and gorditas. What few people realize is that lard actually has less saturated fat than butter. That does not mean it is good to consume lard in large quantities, but for those who see no danger in the occasional pat of butter on pancakes, a few tamales should pose no problems. The main difficulty is that most of our lard is at least partially hydrogenated.

If you are unable to find fresh unhydrogenated lard at a Mexican grocery, you can easily make your own. For small quantities, cut about ½ cup pork fat into very small pieces, place it in a microwave-safe dish, and cover it with good-quality plastic wrap. Microwave it on High, a minute at a time, until most of the fat has rendered and what is left is beginning to turn golden, 2–3 minutes. For large quantities, put the cut-up fat in a 300° oven and pour off the rendered fat about every 5–10 minutes. Virgin coconut oil makes a good substitute for lard in tamales.

MAYONNAISE AND MIRACLE WHIP Mayonnaise has about 100 calories per tablespoon, while Miracle Whip comes in at only 40. And Miracle Whip has only one-third the saturated fat of mayo. While you may not like Miracle Whip as well as mayo, when they are mixed together to prepare something like Thousand Island dressing, which has a number of other spicy ingredients, using at least some Miracle Whip works well for both taste and to create a better nutrition profile. Of course, you could use the low-fat versions of both mayonnaise and Miracle Whip if you like them. To me they eliminate more taste than calories.

NOPALITOS Culinarily speaking, the word *nopal* refers to the paddle of the nopal cactus, genus *Opuntia*, often referred to as prickly pear. The word *nopalitos* is the diminutive form of *nopal* and describes the paddles after they have been sliced or chopped into little pieces. In Mexico the plant, which contains antioxidants and pectin, a soluble fiber, has been used both as food and in indigenous curing for centuries. It is thought to slow the body's absorption of carbohydrates and to lower blood glucose, and for that reason it is considered an ideal food for diabetics. In Mexico it is used to treat Type 2 diabetes. There is growing scientific evidence to support these claims and nopal's ability to lower cholesterol.

The plant can be prepared in many ways, including as a refreshing smoothie; as part of an entrée stew with seafood, poultry, or other items; as a vegetable accompaniment; and as an ingredient in salads and soup. That prickly pears are so nutritious and potentially healing is only half the story. They are also delicious when properly prepared. For those reasons and because so few people know much about them, especially regarding their preparation, this book contains several recipes.

Cooked nopalitos are available in jars or cans in most parts of the country. From the standpoint of taste, they are all right for use in salads but, like canned hominy, they have massive amounts of sodium. The one with the least salt I have found lists 1,460 milligrams of sodium for one ¾-cup serving. To put that into perspective, the Mayo clinic reports that the 2010 Dietary Guidelines for Americans recommends limiting sodium to fewer than 2,300 milligrams a day, or 1,500 milligrams for those who are over fifty-one years old or who have high blood pressure, diabetes, or chronic kidney disease.

Fresh cactus paddles, either whole or sliced, are often available in southwestern supermarkets and in Hispanic markets in other parts of the country, and some varieties have been developed that have almost no thorns. If you find one in a market, take it home and stick the base a couple of inches into a pot filled with a combination of soil and coarse sand and don't water it for two or three weeks. It should soon start sprouting new paddles, and before long you will have an impressive-looking, nutritious plant. Just keep it warm in the winter. If you do grow your own, there is a tip I was given many years ago that appears to work: pick the paddles you plan to use before they have gotten much sun and there will be less of the mucilaginous liquid.

But be aware that not all nopales are tender enough to be palatable. If you live in a part of the country where they grow wild, do take the time to study those sold for consumption before picking your own. You will find that the best ones, bred for eating, have paddles that are usually no more than 8 inches long and 4 inches wide. More important, the best ones will be less than ¼-inch thick.

Whether you use cactus from your garden or from a store, you must first slice off the tough outer perimeter, about ⅛ inch around the entire circumference. This is fairly easy if there are no spines. If there are, you must use a combination of kitchen tongs and gloves to keep from being punctured. You must then remove the spines and nodes they grow from with the end of a paring knife or vegetable peeler. Do leave the rest of the green outer skin intact. In many parts of the country you will be able to buy the cactus already processed to this point, either whole or chopped into nopalitos, and they are certainly worth the small extra cost.

Like okra, cactus paddles contain an unpleasant viscous liquid. Water absorbed by the cactus is converted to this substance because it retards evaporation and helps the plant live in desert conditions. While some people do not find this substance offensive, most do. Fortunately, if cooked properly, nearly all of it can be eliminated. The best way I have found to cook nopalitos for use in stews and side dishes is the one advocated by both Diana Kennedy and Rick Bayless. The nopalitos are fried, often with some onions in a little oil in a covered pot for about five minutes. When the lid is removed you will see that they have released much of the unpleasant substance. To get rid of it, turn the heat to medium-high and continue cooking, uncovered and stirring frequently, until the liquid has evaporated.

To prepare nopalitos for salads, most people simmer them in water for 10 minutes or so and then drain, rinse, and chill them. This removes most, but not all, of the mucus-like liquid. I also did that until I spoke at a Culinary Institute of America workshop, where another presenter, Enrique Olvera, chef and owner of Mexico City's Pujol Restaurant, described a much better and simpler solution. You toss the chopped cactus with salt, leave it in a strainer to drain for about 15 minutes, rinse off the salt, and chill it in ice water. No cooking! I find that the process does leave some of the liquid in the cactus, but the taste is so much fresher that it doesn't matter, at least to me.

There is a similar solution for whole charbroiled nopales, a staple with *barbacoa* and grilled foods in Mexico. You first slice the paddle lengthwise, about every inch, from the rounded top to within about 2 inches of the base. You then have two choices: you can brush the paddles with oil and grill them until tender, or you can salt them for 15 minutes, rinse off the salt, and then oil and grill them. The former leaves a fair amount of the viscous liquid, while the latter removes nearly all of it and produces a delicious result.

When you use nopalitos in smoothies you do not need to do anything but thoroughly rinse the pieces before adding them to the blender.

OLIVE OIL For reasons of both health and taste, this book often calls for olive oil. Wherever it is specified, please use extra-virgin olive oil.

PEPITAS In Mexican cooking, *pepitas* nearly always refers to the green pumpkin seeds that remain after the white hulls have been removed. They are used in stews, sauces, salsas, and as snacks. Their healthy omega-3 fatty acid content is among the highest of any vegetable source, although there is debate as to just how useful it is compared to the omega-3 from sources like salmon and tuna. For snacks and before being incorporated into other dishes, *pepitas* are usually toasted until they pop like popcorn, but not as violently, making them crispy, light, and more flavorful.

PILONCILLO   *Piloncillo* is unrefined cane sugar that comes in very hard cones. It must be grated or chopped and melted, a task that is neither easy nor fun. Instead of using *piloncillo*, I substitute *melao*, which is cane syrup that tastes as close to melted *piloncillo* as it needs to and is available at most Hispanic groceries.

SOUR CREAM   Sour cream is used in many recipes, sometimes as a substitute for high-calorie crema mexicana, Mexico's answer to crème fraîche. Tofutti is a great substitute for the lactose intolerant.

TRUFFLE OIL   A few of the *alta cocina* (upscale cooking) recipes are flavored with a small amount of truffle oil. Truffles are hideously expensive, but, fortunately, a reasonable facsimile of their flavor is available in the form of white truffle oil. Good-quality oil can be found in 3.5-ounce bottles for $18–$30. That may still seem expensive, but a teaspoon or two goes a very long way. After opening the bottle, keep it refrigerated to extend its life.

VINEGAR   Most of the recipes call for rice vinegar because it better mimics the milder vinegars often found in Mexico.

Cooking Techniques

There are some techniques that are particular to Mexican cooking and are used often. Examples include rehydrating dried chiles, roasting and peeling fresh ones, and softening corn tortillas in a little oil so they can be used to make things like enchiladas without cracking or becoming soggy. Rather than repeating the instructions in each recipe, they are included below.

TOASTING DRIED CHILES   Dried chiles are toasted to boost their flavor. The simple process also temporarily softens dried chiles, making them easier to work with.

Heat a skillet over medium heat, place a chile in it, and lightly press the chile into the pan's surface with a spatula. The chile is properly toasted when it just begins to darken and gives off a pleasant roasted aroma, about 15–30 seconds on each side. Thin-skinned chiles such as guajillos require less time than those with thicker skins, like anchos. It is important not to scorch the chiles, so it is better to err on the side of undertoasting.

REHYDRATING DRIED CHILES   To use dried chiles in sauces and salsas, they must first be rehydrated, which is done after toasting them. Remove the stems and seeds, tear the chiles into small pieces, and place them in a bowl. A blender jar also works well, especially if you intend to blend the chiles after rehydrating them. Cover the chiles with hot tap water and leave them for 20–30 minutes.

Some thick-skinned fresh chiles, such as poblanos and Anaheims, need to have their skins removed to prevent them from ruining a dish's texture. This is especially important when making things like *chiles rellenos*, *rajas*, and soups.

The skins must first be blistered. My favorite way is to place them on the grill over a newly lighted mesquite wood fire, which, besides charring the skins, gives them a terrific smoked flavor. You can also place the chiles directly on a lighted gas burner and turn them periodically until the entire exterior is blackened. To make them easier to balance, put a very small barbecue grill directly onto the burner. If you do not have a gas stove you can use a butane torch for small quantities. Simply place the chiles on an outdoor barbecue grill and singe them with the torch until they are blackened. Both these methods will yield chiles that are not so overcooked that they lose their firmness.

If firmness and texture are not important you can put the chiles in a toaster oven and char them with the toast function, turning them as they blister until they are done. It will take longer, and the chiles will be much less firm. This method works well for *rajas* and soups, where firmness is not important.

Although not technically roasting, the chiles can also be placed in a deep fryer at about 350°F and fried until the skins are opaque.

Whatever method you choose, once the skins are blistered, place the chiles in a plastic bag for about 20 minutes to sweat, which will make the skins much easier to remove.

"SOFTENING" CORN TORTILLAS
For Soft Tacos and the Like

Unless they are freshly made, corn tortillas, especially the ones sold in most U.S. supermarkets, become a bit hard and will crack if you try to fold or roll them. In order to make soft tacos or to get flautas ready to fry, the tortillas must first be made pliable. This is done by heating them on a griddle or skillet or wrapping them in a kitchen towel and microwaving them until they are soft and flexible. If you want a toasty texture, use the former. If your tortillas are quite dry, dampen a paper towel with cold water and squeeze as much moisture as possible out of it. Wrap the paper towel around the tortillas to be softened and then either wrap a kitchen towel around the paper towel or put the paper towel–wrapped tortillas in a microwave-safe tortilla warmer. Microwave on High until the tortillas are very flexible and slightly rehydrated, 25–40 seconds.

For Enchiladas

When making enchiladas, the tortillas must not only be softened, they must also be moisture resistant to keep them from becoming soggy. Traditionally, tortillas are immersed in very hot oil for a few seconds then drained on paper towels. The much easier and lower-calorie way to do this is to spray both sides of each tortilla with a little oil, wrap a stack of them in a towel or put them in a microwave-safe tortilla warmer, and heat them in a microwave until they are flexible, 25–40 seconds.

ROASTING TOMATOES   In Mexican cooking, tomatoes are often roasted, which cooks them and creates a very special flavor. This is traditionally done on iron *comales* or in skillets, which involves cooking the tomatoes over medium heat and turning them frequently until they are cooked through and blackened on the outside. I have found it much easier to put the tomatoes in a baking dish or cast iron skillet and place it as close under a broiler as possible. Starting with a cold oven, the process usually takes 15–25 minutes, and you do not have to turn them.

Cooking Equipment

Besides the items that any well-equipped kitchen should have, , there are several items that pertain to either Mexican food or diet that you will find useful.

DIGITAL SCALE   There are many items that do not lend themselves to volume measurement, such as sliced onions, meat, fish, and whole potatoes, and errors can adversely affect both recipes and diet. For example, even lean beef will have about 40 calories per ounce, so an error of just 2 ounces can mean 80 calories. Make that kind of error just once a day and in a year you are off 29,200 calories, enough to gain or lose about seven pounds. With a measuring cup, a lot of guesswork is required, but with an electric food scale there is none at all. Fortunately, there are now many models on the market that perform well, priced from $30 to $60.

LASER THERMOMETER   Serious cooks find these devices invaluable. All you do is point them at a dark surface like that of a skillet, with or without oil, or at something like melting chocolate, and the temperature is immediately visible in the viewfinder. I find them especially useful for making sure my skillet is the right temperature for making tortillas and to judge the exact time to begin frying things like flautas in small amounts of oil. The best ones display temperatures from well below 0°F up to 900°F and can be purchased for $80 to $100.

BLENDER   Just about every kitchen has a blender. The reason I mention it here is that most cooks use ordinary household models. One of the most important tasks in Mexican cooking is puréeing chiles and other foods, such as nuts. Ordinary blenders often leave bits of chile skin, stray seeds, and other items not completely puréed, even after 2–3 minutes. That means you have to put the sauce through a strainer to eliminate them, which is both tedious and messy. And in my experience, most ordinary blenders last but a few years. On the other hand, a commercial-grade blender, such as a Vitamix, will do the job perfectly in less than a minute. They are pricey, but if you shop around (the big-box stores often stock and feature them) you can find a good one for under $400. They are so well made that you may never have to buy another one, and they pay you back every time they make your cooking better and easier.

FOOD PROCESSOR The price of food processors has come so far down that every kitchen should have one. Nothing beats them for grating large amounts of cheese, cutting vegetables in ways that do not demand precision, mixing dough to make flour tortillas and breads, blending salsas where you want some texture, and shredding cooked meat for Mexican fillings, which is easily done with the dough blade.

MOLCAJETE Before the blender and food processor, this ancient stone implement was used to make salsas and to grind spices in Mexico. They are still used, even in Mexican restaurant kitchens, when chefs want their salsas to have just the right texture. Made of volcanic rock, new ones need to be smoothed and cleaned. The best way to do that is to grind several handfuls of rice, washing and rinsing the *molcajete* between grindings. A Japanese mortar and pestle with a rough surface is a decent substitute.

FOOD MILL If you do not choose to buy a commercial-grade blender, you will probably need either a strainer or a food mill. The latter implement, which comes with several blades with different-sized perforations, is perfect for straining out the last bits of seeds and chile skins from blended sauces and is easier to use than a strainer.

SPICE OR COFFEE GRINDER These are relatively cheap and essential for things like powdering annato seeds to make achiote and grinding spices such as whole cumin.

RIDGED GRILL PAN Most people, especially in areas with cold winters, cannot just step outside and fire up a grill whenever they want to. A good substitute, albeit one that does not impart quite as much smoky flavor as even a gas grill, is an iron skillet with ridges on the bottom. Do not get a lightweight one or one with a nonstick surface, as they do not last at the 500°–600°F heat that you need to mimic the real thing.

MEAT TENDERIZER Recipes such as the Imperial Valley Carne Asada (page 172) call for physically tenderizing meat. That can be done by repeatedly stabbing the meat with a fork. A much better option is using one of the spring-loaded devices that plunge rows of narrow, razor-sharp blades into the meat. Jaccard makes at least two models.

Introduction to the Recipes

This book includes the recipes I have collected and used over many years for weight control, health, and—just as important—enjoyment. They come from all branches of Mexican cooking—from the simplest *antojitos mexicanos* (corn and tortilla-based items, such as tacos, enchiladas, and tamales, that in Mexico are often viewed as appetizers or snack foods, but in the United States are often equated with Mexican food itself), to the traditional stews, *moles*, and entrées. And there are dishes from Mexico's exciting new brand of upscale cooking—*alta cocina mexicana*. The latter combines Mexican ingredients and techniques in new ways to create exciting tastes with great eye appeal while retaining the soul-nourishing comfort for which Mexican food is famous.

Although all the recipes are comparatively low in calories, taste and nutritional benefits are equally important priorities. My core assumption is that most people will not make a healthy diet a lifelong endeavor unless they truly enjoy it, and that there are enough naturally good-for-you and delicious Mexican recipes to eliminate the necessity of using any that are not.

As noted in the section on diet and healthy eating, studies have shown that Americans eat portions that are far larger than those eaten by people in other economically advanced countries, such as France and Japan, and that portion size is a major cause of our high levels of obesity. Research also indicates that when we eat delicious food made from quality ingredients with minimal processing, we are satisfied with much smaller portions. For those reasons, my recipe portions are on the moderate side.

NUTRITION ANALYSIS You will see that with each recipe we have included the type of nutrition analysis you now find on packaged foods. The analysis is for one serving. The values are reasonably accurate for most purposes. However, for several reasons, it is difficult to be precise. For example, part of the salt in a can of beans is in the liquid. If you discard the liquid, how much sodium is left in the beans? Several manufacturers reported that they do not have that information.

A similar situation involves marinades. Much of the fat, salt, and other ingredients in a marinade are discarded, but just as obviously, some remain on the meat. Whenever possible I measured the amount of marinade when it was made then measured the amount discarded and assumed the difference remained in the dish. I believe this has produced a reasonable estimate, but one that is not precise. Thus, for those of you for whom the content of one ingredient or another is of critical importance, the calculations in some instances may not be accurate enough for your purposes. In that case, you need to make your own determinations.

You will find that many of the recipes have more than the 30 percent fat from calories often used as a guideline. There are two reasons for that. First, fat is very important in terms of taste and mouth-feel, which together create much of the pleasure related to eating. This, in turn, means that we will be more inclined to make the dish a permanent part of our diets. Second, recent studies indicate that overeating carbohydrates may cause more cardiac problems than eating too much fat, even saturated fat.

Like nearly everything else, the key words are "overeating" and "too much," for it is becoming clear that moderate portions of well-balanced meals are far more healthful than large portions of some low-fat items. And you will discover that in most cases where fat exceeds 30 percent of calories, it comes from healthy extra-virgin olive oil. In any case, if fat is a serious consideration, an alternative to not trying a particular recipe is to minimize your fat intake at other meals or, of course, to use less than is specified.

The following table compares the nutritional content of 1 tablespoon of various fats. It is interesting that lard, which is often thought to be the worst of the bunch, actually has less saturated fat and cholesterol than butter. (Note: The Smart Balance numbers are for Smart Balance made with extra-virgin olive oil.)

It is the same for salt. My use of salt in recipes tends to be on the moderate side, but there are some foods that, for most people, just need more salt than others, such as salsas. In those situations I either limit the portions or make up for the excessive sodium by minimizing it elsewhere in my diet. Of course, you can simply use less salt than specified.

NUTRITIONAL CONTENT OF 1 TABLESPOON OF VARIOUS FATS

	Butter	Lard	Coconut oil (extra virgin)	Duck fat	Olive oil (extra virgin)	Canola Oil	Smart Balance butter substitute
Calories	100.00	120.00	120.00	110.00	130.00	120.00	60.00
Total fat (g)	11.52	12.80	13.00	12.77	14.00	14.00	7.00
Saturated fat (g)	7.29	5.02	13.00	4.25	1.96	1.03	2.00
Mono fat (g)	2.98	5.77	0.00	6.31	10.78	8.86	3.00
Poly fat (g)	0.43	1.43	0.00	1.65	1.26	3.94	2.00
Trans-fatty acids (g)	0.47	0.00	0.00	0.00	0.00	0.06	0.00
Cholesterol (mg)	30.53	12.16	0.00	12.80	0.00	0.00	0.00

Most of the recipes have under 450 calories. I included the few that have more than that because they are especially delicious or their ingredients are particularly healthy. Since there are many very low-calorie items, it is easy to combine them with the few that are higher to get a satisfactory average.

AUTHENTICITY AND SOURCE Some may ask if these recipes are authentic. In previous books my goal was to chronicle recipes from various aspects of Mexican cooking. In doing so, I tried to prepare them in the original manner with the original ingredients whenever possible. In this book, the objective is to provide delicious Mexican recipes to help people live healthier lives. My experience is that many people either do not like to cook as much as I do or they lack the time. Therefore, to make the book useful to the widest possible audience, in some recipes I use shortcuts. At the same time, I have been careful to advocate nothing that would materially alter the authentic flavor of a recipe.

Readers often wonder where the recipes come from. I have sampled virtually all of them in restaurants, food stalls, or private homes during the last forty years. When I decide to work on a recipe, I first find as many versions of it as I can in my library of over 300 Spanish-language Mexican cookbooks, paying special attention to the descriptions, ingredients, and preparation instructions. I then make the dish, guided by both my memory and the reference material. Once I get it to the point that it has the right taste and nutrition profile, I prepare a final draft. Whenever feasible, I list the primary sources used to adapt the recipe. A very few recipes were created entirely by me, usually for restaurant clients.

SUGGESTIONS ON USING THE RECIPES Here are some of the ways I have learned to use the recipes in this book to produce meals that are both easy and healthy.

As mentioned in the introduction to *Antojitos Mexicanos*, to have anything from snacks to entire meals available in just minutes, all you need to do is make one or more of the fillings and salsas. Have some tortillas and, ideally, some ripe avocados and, possibly, some rice and beans on hand. Careful use of a microwave will enable you to produce anything from a taco to several entrées within 5 minutes.

Many of the recipes, including the soups and stews, and even some of the broiled meats and poultry, can be prepared in advance and reheated later. Since most of the recipes are designed to serve four, if you are serving two, one recipe will yield two extra meals. And since most of the recipes can be doubled if you have a large enough pot, you can make enough to refrigerate or freeze for future meals. Think how much better you will eat in terms of both taste and nutrition than if you bought frozen dinners.

One of the best ways to entertain is a *parrillada*, which is a mixed-grill cookout party that is especially popular in northern Mexico. Prepare at least two salsas and heat some tortillas, beans, and/or rice. Just before your guests arrive, make some guacamole and have some items such as beef, pork, chicken, and shrimp ready to grill. You can also have a vegetarian *parrillada*, where you grill things like portobello mushrooms, eggplant, squash, onions, and corn. Grill the foods you choose and serve them piled on a large platter for your guests to help themselves, accompanied by the tortillas, salsas, guacamole, beans, and rice. Grilled mangoes make a particularly delicious and festive dessert.

¡Buen provecho!

DRINKS

MEXICANS ENJOY a great variety of drinks, and many of them are extremely nutritious. Although a few popular alcoholic beverages are included here, the emphasis is on nonalcoholic.

Low-Calorie Cactus Smoothie

1–2 servings

PER SERVING | 120 calories | 2 g protein
27 g carbohydrates | 0 g total fat
(0 g saturated) | 0 mg cholesterol
1 g fiber | 21 g sugar | 10 mg sodium

This very low-calorie drink is a terrific way to consume healthy nopal cactus. What makes it especially useful is that when nopalitos are blended raw, you get none of the viscous liquid that for most people is unpleasant and that, when the cactus is cooked, must be eliminated. If you like things tart, try the drink without the optional agave nectar, but even with it the drink is still quite low in calories.

INGREDIENTS

½ cup cleaned and diced cactus paddle pieces
1 cup orange juice, pomegranate juice, or another juice
Small handful of ice

DIRECTIONS

Rinse the cactus pieces thoroughly under cold running water and put them and the juice and ice in a blender. Blend until thoroughly liquefied, 1–2 minutes.

Atole

4 servings

PER SERVING | 240 calories
14 g protein | 44 g carbohydrates
1.5 g total fat (0 g saturated)
5 mg cholesterol | 1 g fiber
30 g sugar | 250 mg sodium

Atoles are drinks or gruels made with prepared corn masa or corn flour. In pre-Hispanic times, atoles came in untold variations and were used in numerous ways—for breakfast, as a nourishing snack, and as beverages to accompany meals—and they were served both hot and cold. Originally made with water or a combination of water and various juices, they are also delicious made with milk. When chocolate is added, the drink is called Champurrado, which I think makes a more interesting version of hot chocolate.

Atoles are a perfect vehicle for creativity. You can make them thicker—to Cream of Wheat consistency—by adding fruits or nuts, or you can make them with juices. Here is a basic recipe, followed by one for Champurrado. Together, I hope they will serve as a basis from which you will create your own versions. If you use milk, be sure to employ a large pot in order to prevent it from boiling over when it first comes to a boil.

INGREDIENTS

½ cup corn flour, such as Maseca

¼ teaspoon ground cinnamon, preferably *canela*

⅛ teaspoon salt

5 cups nonfat milk or water

4 tablespoons agave nectar

1 teaspoon vanilla extract

DIRECTIONS

Put the corn flour in a large pot with the cinnamon and salt. Slowly stir in the milk or water until the corn flour has dissolved completely. Add the agave nectar and vanilla, bring to a boil, and cook at a low simmer for 5 minutes, stirring constantly to keep it from clumping and sticking to the bottom of the pot.

Champurrado

CHOCOLATE ATOLE

4 servings. Nutrition information is based on using nonfat milk.

PER SERVING | 310 calories
15 g protein | 51 g carbohydrates
7 g total fat (3.5 g saturated)
5 mg cholesterol | 3 g fiber
34 g sugar | 250 mg sodium

I like the amount of chocolate specified here, but it still tastes quite good with half the amount—and even better with another ounce.

INGREDIENTS

Atole (page 24)

2 ounces 70%-cacao-content chocolate

DIRECTIONS

Add the chocolate to the *atole* after it has simmered for 4 minutes. Cook for 1 minute more, stirring until the chocolate has melted.

Aguas Frescas

4 servings

PER SERVING | 70 calories | 0 g protein
18 g carbohydrates | 0 g total fat
(0 g saturated) | 0 mg cholesterol
0 g fiber | 17 g sugar | 5 mg sodium

Aguas frescas means "fresh waters" or "cool waters," which is a nearly perfect description. And they are easy to make: just blend together some fruit, lime juice, water, and a little sugar or sugar substitute, and you have a nutritious and delicious drink. They are especially suitable when made in bulk and served at parties. Of course, a little tequila, rum, or wine can be included. Aguas Frescas can be made with most fruits and combinations of them. Some of the most popular are watermelon, pineapple, cantaloupe, papaya, and mango. Fruits like oranges and grapefruits that have bitter-tasting, pithy fibers are less successful, although their juices make nice additions. Aguas Frescas that are made with tart fruits, such as tamarind, or those made without real fruit, such as jamaica, require too much sweetener to fit our needs. Although I use the easy-to-remember proportions listed below, I hope you will experiment, perhaps by increasing the fruit-to-water ratio, and with your own fruit combinations.

INGREDIENTS

2 cups fresh fruit
1–2 tablespoons freshly squeezed lime juice
2 cups water
2–4 tablespoons agave nectar or a sugar substitute
1 cup crushed ice

DIRECTIONS

Purée the fruit, lime juice, water, and agave nectar in a blender. Strain into a pitcher and add the ice.

Horchata de Melón

HORCHATA MADE
WITH CANTALOUPE

About 4 twelve-ounce servings

PER SERVING | 70 calories | 1 g protein
18 g carbohydrates | 0 g total fat
(0 g saturated) | 0 mg cholesterol
1 g fiber | 16 g sugar | 25 mg sodium

Horchata was originally brought to Mexico from Spain and, like most other imports, was immediately Mexicanized, at least to some extent. Most Horchata is made with soaked raw rice that is blended with milk and cinnamon and sometimes a few almonds. While this version is filled with natural ingredients, the rice adds a lot of calories (about 250 for 12 ounces) and carbohydrates. Also, unlike the drinks made with fruit, Horchata tastes a bit chalky unless you add a fair amount of agave nectar, sugar, or sugar substitute.

Fortunately, other versions are made with melon and melon seeds that are even better and much more healthy. The following refreshing and delicious Horchata is my favorite. If you are really interested in keeping the nutrition counts healthy, you may want to try leaving out both the lime juice and the sugar to see how you like it. As written here, a 12-ounce portion has only 70 calories, more than a third less than most fresh juices.

2 tablespoons freshly squeezed lime juice (optional)

1 ripe cantaloupe, approximately 2 pounds, yielding
    about 1 pound of pure fruit and seeds, 2½ cups

2½ cups water

2 tablespoons agave nectar or sugar substitute (optional)

½ teaspoon vanilla extract

DIRECTIONS

Put the lime juice, if using, 1 cup water, and the fruit and seeds in a blender and purée. Add the rest of the water, the sweetener, if using, and the vanilla and blend to mix well. Strain the Horchata into a pitcher and chill or serve over ice.

Margarita

1 serving

PER SERVING | 250 calories | 0 g protein
12 g carbohydrates | 0 g total fat
(0 g saturated) | 0 mg cholesterol
0 g fiber | 12 g sugar | 0 mg sodium

I make the following Margarita more than any other, probably because the recipe is so easy to remember. The drink can be served up, on the rocks, or frozen.

INGREDIENTS

1½ ounces tequila

1½ ounces freshly squeezed lime juice

1½ ounces triple sec, Cointreau, or Grand Marnier

Handful of ice

DIRECTIONS

To serve up. Place all the ingredients in a cocktail shaker, shake, and strain into a Margarita glass.

To serve on the rocks. Place all the ingredients in a cocktail shaker, shake, and pour into a large glass.

To serve frozen. Place all the ingredients in a blender, blend until puréed, and pour into a large Margarita glass.

Sangría

About 12 six-ounce servings

PER SERVING | 180 calories | 0 g protein
14 g carbohydrates | 0 g total fat
(0 g saturated) | 0 mg cholesterol
0 g fiber | 9 g sugar | 10 mg sodium

Originally from Spain, there are many versions of this alcoholic fruit punch. The following is my favorite, but beware, as it packs a punch— a real punch of a different sort. I served it at a signing for my first book, and it may have been at least partially responsible for the sale of over 150 books that evening!

INGREDIENTS

1 quart port
1 cup brandy
1½ cups orange juice
Juice of 2 limes
2 cups club soda
2 oranges, sliced

DIRECTIONS

In a large punch bowl, combine the port, brandy, orange juice, and lime juice. Just before serving, stir in the club soda and add the orange slices and enough ice (preferably in a large block) to chill the contents.

Sangrita

About 3 cups, about 12 quarter-cup chasers to be served with chilled shots of tequila

PER SERVING | 45 calories | 1 g protein
10 g carbohydrates | 0 g total fat
(0 g saturated) | 0 mg cholesterol
1 g fiber | 7 g sugar | 200 mg sodium

Sangrita is a nonalcoholic concoction whose main use is as a chaser to tequila, and that combination is probably the most popular way to drink tequila in Mexico. Some people add tomato sauce, and if you like Bloody Marys you might like it that way. If so, just add 1 cup tomato juice to the recipe, or to your taste. Some mixologists add a little onion and/or celery to be blended with the other ingredients.

INGREDIENTS

2 medium-sized ancho chiles, toasted and rehydrated (pages 15–16)
2½ cups fresh orange juice
3½ tablespoons grenadine
1 teaspoon salt

DIRECTIONS

Put all the ingredients in a blender and purée. Strain and chill the mixture before serving.

TORTILLAS

CORN TORTILLAS arrived on the Mexican culinary scene around AD 500, which is when archeologists date the first clay *comales* used to cook them. When the Spanish arrived in warm and humid southern Mexico, they were unable to successfully grow wheat from the seeds they had brought, so they adopted tortillas as their basic bread. Later, when they found that wheat thrived in northern Mexico, instead of using it to make bread, they invented a new kind of tortilla. Today, chefs are experimenting with combining corn and flour to create new and interesting tortilla varieties.

Corn tortillas can be successfully reheated in a microwave when wrapped in a kitchen towel or placed in a tortilla warmer (see the instructions on page 16). If they are particularly dry, use a slightly dampened towel. On the other hand, a few seconds too long in a microwave will cause flour tortillas to become tough and rubbery. They are best reheated in a hot ungreased skillet or on a griddle.

Corn
Tortillas

8 tortillas

PER SERVING | 50 calories | 2 g protein
10 g carbohydrates | 0 g total fat
(0 g saturated) | 0 mg cholesterol
1 g fiber | 0 g sugar | 0 mg sodium

Very good corn tortillas can be made at home, but not nearly as easily as flour tortillas. You might well ask, "Why would I want to make them when my supermarket sells them?" There are several reasons. First, a freshly made corn tortilla has a special taste and texture that lasts but a short time. Second, traditional tortillas contain only corn, traces of the lime used to remove the skin from the kernels, and water. Unfortunately, without loads of chemical preservatives, corn tortillas degrade quickly, and that does not suit supermarkets' needs. Check the ingredients on a package of supermarket tortillas and you will see what I mean. If you cannot make your own, look for a tortilla factory that minimizes chemical preservatives.

If you can get freshly prepared nixtamal from a tortilla factory, by all means use it. However, most of us must use dried corn flour to make the masa. My favorite brand is Maseca, which lists the ingredients as "corn treated with lime." Once you mix the water into the flour, knead it for at least 1 minute, then be sure to let it rest for a half hour, covered with plastic wrap so it will be completely hydrated. You should then knead it again, adding some cold water to get it to the perfect consistency, which is about the same as very smooth modeling clay. If there is too little liquid, the tortillas will fall apart; if there is too much, the dough will tend to stick, and the tortillas will be gummy. A little practice will give you a feel for the right balance.

Some cooks replace about 1 tablespoon of the corn flour with 1 tablespoon of all-purpose flour per cup of corn flour in the recipe to better mimic the elasticity of tortillas made from fresh masa.

One of the biggest mistakes novices make is to cook corn tortillas over insufficient heat. Like flour tortillas, they are best cooked at between 425° and 450°F (yet another reason to have a laser thermometer).

You will need a hand-operated tortilla press and some plastic to keep the dough from sticking to it. I think plastic wrap is a little too thin, so I cut pieces from small garbage bags to be slightly larger than the surface of the press. If possible, cook the tortillas on an ungreased iron plancha (griddle) or skillet.

INGREDIENTS

1 cup corn flour for tortillas
⅔ cup warm water, plus a little cold water

DIRECTIONS

Make the masa. Put the corn flour in a bowl and stir the warm water into the flour with a wooden spoon. Work the dough with your hands and knead it for about 1 minute. Allow the dough to rest, covered with plastic wrap, for 30 minutes.

Finish the dough. Add about ½ tablespoon cold water to the bowl and work it into the dough with your hands. Knead the dough, adding only enough water to get a silky smooth, clay-like consistency. Separate the dough into 8 pieces and roll them into smooth little balls.

Preheat your skillet or griddle to 425°–450°F.

Press the dough. While the skillet is heating, lay a piece of plastic on the bottom of the tortilla press. Place a dough ball just off center, toward the press's hinge, flatten the dough slightly with the palm of your hand, and put another piece of plastic on top of it. Press firmly on the handle to flatten the dough to about 5 inches in diameter.

Transfer the dough to the hot skillet. Once you get the masa's consistency down, this is the most difficult part of the process. Carefully peel the top piece of plastic off the flattened dough. If you are right-handed, use it to put the dough, plastic side down, on your left hand. Hold your right hand palm up and spread your fingers slightly. With your left hand, carefully place the uncooked tortilla, dough side down, on the palm of your right hand. Carefully pull off the second piece of plastic.

With your knuckles facing down, pass your hand about an inch over the hot surface of the skillet, tilting your hand slightly so that the trailing edge of the dough touches the skillet's surface. At that point, continue sweeping your right palm close to the surface and, as you do so, turn your right palm upward to allow gravity to release the dough onto the hot surface. This is a bit tricky to learn, but once mastered, it is quite easy. You may want to practice by cutting some paper to tortilla size and releasing it onto a table or another flat surface.

Cook the tortillas. Cook the tortilla for about a minute, at which time the bottom should be developing brown spots. Turn the tortilla and cook it another minute on the other side. The tortilla should begin to puff as the dough cooks through. You can facilitate this by "tickling it": lightly stroking the dough with the sharp edge of your spatula. Wrap the cooked tortillas in a towel or put them into a tortilla warmer.

Flour Tortillas

12 tortillas

PER SERVING | 100 calories | 2 g protein
16 g carbohydrates | 2.5 g total fat
(0.5 g saturated) | 0 mg cholesterol
1 g fiber | 0 g sugar | 20 mg sodium

Unlike corn tortillas, flour tortillas are very easy to make at home. The only problem is that they are often made with over-processed white flour. You can always use some whole wheat flour combined with unbleached white flour, but most people find that changes the nature of what they wanted in the first place. However, using unbleached white all-purpose flour with a butter substitute or a small amount of extra-virgin olive oil instead of the usual lard, butter, or shortening does improve the nutrition profile without significantly affecting the result.

Most flour in Mexico is softer than ours, which means it has a lower protein content, which in turn means that the dough is less elastic and thus easier to shape. It also produces tortillas that are softer and less rubbery. To make up for the difference in protein, I substitute up to half low-protein unbleached cake flour to the recipe, but you can certainly make them entirely with all-purpose flour or vary the proportions to suit yourself. The recipe can be made with as little as 1 tablespoon extra-virgin olive oil, canola oil, or coconut oil, but my favorite option is to use 4 tablespoons of butter substitute. The extra butter substitute adds a lot of flavor and only about 10 calories per tortilla.

The recipe makes 12 medium-thick tortillas about 6–7 inches in diameter. To make thicker Tex-Mex-style tortillas, add ½ teaspoon baking powder to the flour and salt, divide the dough into 10 pieces, and roll them to a diameter of 6–7 inches. To make very thin tortillas, such as those found in Arizona and California, divide the dough into 16 pieces and roll them to 7–7½ inches.

To make tortillas for burritos, divide the dough into 8 pieces and roll to a diameter of about 9 inches. This makes a fairly small burrito, but that is about the maximum size for home griddles and skillets. If your equipment permits larger sizes, divide the dough into 6 pieces and roll out to about 12 inches.

To make a quick version of Pan Árabe to serve with Tacos Árabes (page 130), replace ¼ cup all-purpose flour with ¼ cup whole wheat flour in the basic Flour Tortilla recipe.

INGREDIENTS

1 cup all-purpose flour

1 cup cake flour

½ teaspoon salt

⅔ cup hot tap water

¼ cup Smart Balance with extra-virgin olive oil, or 1 tablespoon extra-virgin olive, canola, or coconut oil

Make the dough. The easiest way to make the dough is in a food processor, but it can also be mixed by hand in a bowl, preferably with a wooden spoon. Put the flours and salt in a food processor fitted with the steel blade. Heat the hot water and butter substitute or oil in a microwave-safe container until the butter is just melted or, if using oil, for about 30 seconds. Turn on the processor and slowly pour the liquid through the feed tube into the flour until the dough just comes together.

Remove the dough and knead it by hand until it is very smooth. Divide the dough into 12 equal balls (or whatever number you decide on; see above) and roll them in your hands until they are smooth. Place them on a plate or countertop, cover with a damp kitchen towel, and let them rest for 20 minutes. This allows the gluten to relax and makes them easier to roll.

Form the tortillas. Except for burrito-sized tortillas, it is easiest to roll the dough with a shorter-than-usual rolling pin. A French-style rolling pin (one piece of shaped wood) about 12–14 inches long is ideal.

Dust your work surface with a little flour, place one of the dough balls on it, and flatten it with your hand. Starting at the bottom of the dough, roll straight up and then back. Give the dough a quarter turn and again roll straight up and down. After four turns, flip the dough over and repeat the process, adding more flour to the work surface if necessary, until the tortilla is 6–7 inches in diameter.

Cook the tortillas. When making tortillas, temperature matters. The ideal is between 425° and 450°F, and the best way to check the temperature is with a laser thermometer, but be aware that they are accurate only on dark surfaces. I use an iron griddle over medium heat.

Place a formed piece of dough on the preheated surface and leave it until it begins to puff and get brown spots on the bottom, 20–30 seconds. Turn the tortilla and continue cooking until it is just cooked through, 10–15 seconds. Wrap the cooked tortillas in a towel or put them into a tortilla warmer.

Hybrid Tortillas

Chefs like to experiment, and the results can be rewarding. In this case, the outcome is a combination of corn and flour tortillas with a blend of tastes and textures that is quite interesting. They are definitely worth trying and very easy to make.

12 tortillas

PER SERVING | 90 calories | 2 g protein
15 g carbohydrates | 2.5 g total fat
(0.5 g saturated) | 0 mg cholesterol
1 g fiber | 0 g sugar | 25 mg sodium

INGREDIENTS

1⅓ cups all-purpose flour
⅔ cup corn flour for tortillas, such as Maseca
½ teaspoon salt
⅔ cup hot tap water
¼ cup Smart Balance with extra-virgin olive oil, or
    1 tablespoon extra-virgin olive, canola, or coconut oil

DIRECTIONS

Make the dough. The easiest way to make the dough is in a food processor, but it can also be mixed by hand in a bowl, preferably with a wooden spoon. Put the flours and salt in a food processor fitted with the steel blade. Heat the hot water and butter substitute or oil in a microwave-safe container until the butter is just melted or, if using oil, about 30 seconds. Turn on the processor and slowly pour the liquid through the feed tube into the flour until the dough just comes together, 10–15 seconds.

Remove the dough and knead it by hand until it is very smooth. Divide the dough into 12 equal balls and roll them in your hands until they are smooth. Place them on a plate or countertop, cover with a damp towel, and let them rest for 20 minutes. This allows the gluten to relax and makes them easier to roll.

Form the tortillas. Dust your work surface with a little flour, place one of the dough balls on it, and flatten it with your hand. Starting at the bottom of the dough, roll straight up and then back. Give the dough a quarter turn and again roll straight up and down. After four turns, flip the dough over and repeat the process, adding more flour to the work surface if necessary, until the tortilla is 6–7 inches in diameter.

Cook the tortillas. When making tortillas, temperature matters. The ideal is between 425° and 450°F, and the best way to check the temperature is with a laser thermometer, but be aware that they are accurate only on dark surfaces. I use an iron griddle over medium heat.

Place a formed piece of dough on the preheated surface and leave it until it begins to puff and get brown spots on the bottom, 20–30 seconds. Turn the tortilla and continue cooking until it is just cooked through, 10–15 seconds. Wrap the cooked tortillas in a towel or put them into a tortilla warmer.

SALSAS & RELISHES

EVEN PEOPLE who dine often in Mexican restaurants in the United States miss the true variety and enjoyment of Mexican salsas. The principal reason is that to minimize food costs restaurateurs make buckets full of it, usually partially from canned ingredients. Rarely are we exposed to the delights of salsas made from fresh ingredients, often roasted individually before being combined and processed to just the right texture, as called for in most of the following recipes.

Salsa Fresca

About 1 cup. Nutrition information is for 1 tablespoon.

PER SERVING | 5 calories | 0 g protein
1 g carbohydrates | 0 g total fat
(0 g saturated) | 0 mg cholesterol
0 g fiber | 1 g sugar | 75 mg sodium

This is close to my favorite all-purpose salsa. It is found in open-air markets all over Mexico and is best made with a meat grinder. If you don't have one, you can use a food processor with the added water suggested in the recipe. Be sure to use Roma tomatoes, as they are less watery and stand up better to grinding than regular tomatoes. They also keep their color better.

INGREDIENTS

4 ounces tomatillos, husked, rinsed, dried, and cut into ¾-inch pieces
6 ounces Roma tomatoes, cut into ¾-inch pieces
¼-ounce serrano chile (about 1¼ inches) long, cut into ⅓-inch pieces
¼ cup loosely packed, roughly chopped cilantro
¼ cup very finely chopped white onion
½ teaspoon salt
¼ cup water (optional)

DIRECTIONS

Grind or chop the ingredients. If you have a meat grinder, grind together into a bowl the tomatillos, tomatoes, chile, and cilantro. Stir in the onion and salt. If you are using a food processor, put the tomatillos, tomatoes, chile, and cilantro into the work bowl, add ¼ cup water, and pulse until everything is finely chopped (as if it had been put through a meat grinder). Stir in the onions and salt.

Salsa de Tomatillos Asados

ROASTED TOMATILLO SALSA

About 1¼ cups. Nutrition information is for 1 tablespoon.

PER SERVING | 15 calories | 0 g protein
3 g carbohydrates | 0 g total fat
(0 g saturated) | 0 mg cholesterol
0 g fiber | 2 g sugar | 115 mg sodium

This salsa has a bold, earthy texture and a flavor that is perfect with grilled foods. I used to roast the ingredients under a broiler, because roasting whole tomatillos the authentic way—in a dry skillet—took too long and was too much trouble. Then I saw a recipe from Rick Bayless that called for cutting the tomatillos in half and dry roasting them in the skillet with the other ingredients. That technique pares the time down to about 8 minutes and produces an excellent result. Also, the agave nectar does a great job of balancing the naturally tart flavor of tomatillos. You can make the salsa in a food processor or blender, but I prefer the processor because it allows you to pulse the ingredients with more accuracy. Of course, you can also use a molcajete, which will give you the perfect earthy texture.

INGREDIENTS

12 ounces tomatillos, husked, rinsed, dried, and cut in half
1 medium to large serrano pepper
3 cloves garlic, unpeeled
½-inch slice white onion
1 teaspoon salt

1 teaspoon canola oil
1½ teaspoons agave nectar
2 tablespoons roughly chopped cilantro, or to taste

DIRECTIONS

Roast the vegetables. Heat a skillet over medium to medium-high heat and put in the tomatillos, cut side down. Add the serrano pepper, garlic, and onion slice and cook until the tomatillos are blackened on the bottom, 3½–4 minutes. Turn the tomatillos, pepper, garlic, and onion, and cook until the tomatillos are blackened on the other side, 3½–4 minutes. Put the tomatillos, serrano, and onion in a food processor. When the garlic has cooled enough to handle, peel and add to the processor.

    Finish the salsa. Add the salt, oil, agave nectar, and cilantro to the processor and pulse until well combined and with the texture you want.

Roasted-Tomato and Pumpkin Seed Salsa

About 2½ cups. Nutrition information is for 1 tablespoon.

PER SERVING | 15 calories | 1 g protein
1 g carbohydrates | 1 g total fat
(0 g saturated) | 0 mg cholesterol
0 g fiber | 1 g sugar | 60 mg sodium

Made mostly with tomatoes and pumpkin seeds, one of the few fruits or vegetables that contain omega-3 fatty acids in meaningful quantities, it is hard to find a more nutritious salsa than this one. That it is also delicious and versatile makes it a winner. It makes a fine dip with tortilla chips, a salsa for tacos and the like, an enchilada sauce, and an accompaniment for everything from eggs to poultry. It is especially delicious heated and used to smother grilled or sautéed pork or chicken to create a simple and delicious mole.

INGREDIENTS

3 or 4 tomatoes, for a total of about 1½ pounds
1 medium to large serrano chile
½-inch slice of white onion
2 cloves garlic, peeled
½ cup toasted and ground pumpkin seeds (*pepitas*)
    (from ⅔ cup raw hulled pumpkin seeds)
1 teaspoon salt, or to taste

DIRECTIONS

Cook the vegetables. Put the tomatoes and chile on a baking sheet as close to your broiler as possible and broil until the tomatoes have softened and just begin to char, 10–15 minutes. Add the onion and garlic and continue cooking until the onion is a bit charred and the garlic is soft, 5–10 more minutes. Make sure the tomatoes are cooked through and quite soft. Remove the vegetables from the oven, put them in a food processor, add the salt, and process until the sauce is smooth. ▶▶

Toast and grind the pumpkin seeds and finish the salsa. While the vegetables are broiling, heat a nonstick skillet over medium heat and toast the pumpkin seeds, stirring or shaking often, until most of them have popped (like popcorn, but not nearly as violently). Don't let them scorch. Grind the toasted seeds to a powder in a spice or coffee grinder. Add ½ cup of the ground seeds and the salt to the processor and pulse with the other ingredients until everything is well combined.

Jalisco-style Pico de Gallo

About 3 cups. Nutrition information is for 1 tablespoon.

PER SERVING | 5 calories | 0 g protein
1 g carbohydrates | 0 g total fat
(0 g saturated) | 0 mg cholesterol
0 g fiber | 1 g sugar | 5 mg sodium

In the United States we usually think of pico de gallo as the combination of chopped tomato, onion, fresh green chiles, and cilantro that often accompanies fajitas. And that's true in much of Mexico, as well, especially in the north. However, in the state of Jalisco, pico de gallo is a relish of sweet fruits, cucumber, jícama, and other ingredients, seasoned with chile sauce or powder and lime juice. It makes a wonderful appetizer, fruit salad, or accompaniment to broiled foods. It also goes well with a plate of tortilla chips set beside a chilled glass of tequila. It is always best to use fresh ingredients but, for convenience, feel free to substitute canned pineapple or mandarin oranges. If you do use canned ingredients, try to use those that are not canned in sugar syrup. If that is unavoidable, rinse the fruits off before chopping them.

INGREDIENTS

½ cup peeled, seeded, and chopped cucumber, ½-inch pieces
½ cup mango, chopped into ½-inch pieces
½ cup pineapple, chopped into ½-inch pieces
½ cup orange or tangerine segments, cut into ½-inch pieces
½ cup peeled and finely chopped jícama
½ cup thinly sliced red onion
2 tablespoons freshly squeezed lime juice
⅛ heaping teaspoon salt
1 teaspoon pure ancho chile powder, or ½ teaspoon powder
    made from chile de árbol

DIRECTIONS

Make the salsa. Combine everything except the salt and chile powder. Stir in the salt and chile powder and refrigerate for ½ hour to let the flavors meld before serving.

Fresh Tomatillo Salsa

About 1¼ cups. Nutrition information is for 1 tablespoon.

PER SERVING | 5 calories | 0 g protein
1 g carbohydrates | 0 g total fat
(0 g saturated) | 0 mg cholesterol
0 g fiber | 1 g sugar | 130 mg sodium

This is the freshest-tasting and most visually appealing version of tomatillo salsa. It is also the easiest to prepare. I adapted it from one presented by the great chef and Mexican food expert Ricardo Muñoz in Verde en la cocina mexicana. *It can also be used to make a delicious seafood cocktail. For a great alternative to guacamole, add one large chopped avocado to the salsa. It is delicious, and the avocado will stay green for a day or two.*

INGREDIENTS

¾ **pound fresh tomatillos, husked, rinsed, dried, and cut into quarters**
1 medium-sized serrano chile, stem removed, finely chopped
3 tablespoons chopped white onion
3 tablespoons chopped cilantro
1 heaping teaspoon salt

DIRECTIONS

Make the salsa. Place all the ingredients in a blender and pulse just until the sauce is thick and chunky but not completely puréed.

Salsa Ranchera

RANCH-STYLE SALSA

About 2 cups. Nutrition information is for 1 tablespoon.

PER SERVING | 10 calories | 0 g protein
1 g carbohydrates | 0 g total fat
(0 g saturated) | 0 mg cholestero
0 g fiber | 1 g sugar | 35 mg sodium

Salsa Ranchera comes in many different forms. Sometimes it is made with chopped tomatoes, onions, and fresh chiles. Other recipes, such as this one, which I adapted from one by food writer Kippy Nigh, are made with dried chiles. This version is relatively mild and is particularly suitable for serving over eggs, pork, or poultry. It is also good on chiles rellenos.

INGREDIENTS

1 large guajillo chile, stemmed, seeded, toasted, and rehydrated (pages 15–16), ½ cup of the soaking water reserved
1 pound tomatoes (about 2 medium to large), roasted (page 17)
1 tablespoon extra-virgin olive oil
1½ cups chopped white onion
1 clove garlic, minced
½ teaspoon salt

DIRECTIONS

Blend the tomatoes and chiles. Place the chiles, tomatoes, and the ½ cup chile soaking water in a blender and purée completely, 1–2 minutes. If not completely smooth, put the ingredients through the fine blade of a food mill or press them through a strainer.

   Sauté the onions and garlic. Heat a large saucepan over medium to medium-low heat, add the oil and onions, and sauté them until they are soft but not browned, 4–5 minutes. Add the garlic and cook another minute. ▸▸

Finish the salsa. Pour the tomatoes and chiles into the saucepan with the onion and garlic and stir in the salt. Bring to a simmer and cook for 5–10 minutes, or until the sauce holds together. If it becomes too thick, add a little more water.

Mango Salsa

About 1¾ cups. Nutrition information is for 1 tablespoon.

PER SERVING | 5 calories | 0 g protein
2 g carbohydrates | 0 g total fat
(0 g saturated) | 0 mg cholesterol
0 g fiber | 1 g sugar | 0 mg sodium

Quick, easy, and delicious, this salsa is ideal with seafood, poultry, and pork.

INGREDIENTS

1½ cups diced mango (about 2 large mangoes)
⅓ cup finely chopped red onion
2 tablespoons chopped cilantro
1 teaspoon freshly squeezed lime juice

DIRECTIONS

Make the salsa. Mix all the ingredients in a bowl and refrigerate for 1 hour to let the flavors meld.

Salsa Habanero

HABANERO SALSA

About ¾ cup. Nutrition information is for 1 tablespoon.

PER SERVING | 25 calories | 0 g protein
6 g carbohydrates | 0 g total fat
(0 g saturated) | 0 mg cholesterol
0 g fiber | 5 g sugar | 350 mg sodium

In Mexico's Yucatán, cooks often leave a whole or halved habanero chile in their sauces as they cook and then remove and discard the chile to minimize the heat. This one is made with puréed habaneros and garlic and relies on the acid in the pineapple juice and vinegar, as well as removal of the potent chile veins, to moderate the heat. Nevertheless, most Mexicans would use only a very small amount, perhaps a small spoonful, rubbed over fish or meat. In such small portions the salsa is delicious and provides a very satisfying heat. It also minimizes the otherwise high salt content of a full tablespoon to something much more reasonable. The sauce is very simple to make, but be sure you do not blend the ingredients until the liquid has cooled. The steam from hot liquid can blow the top off a blender and cause serious burns, in this case from both the stove's heat and the chiles.

INGREDIENTS

5 habanero chiles, seeds and veins removed, roughly chopped
½ cup cider vinegar
½ cup pineapple juice
4 cloves garlic, unpeeled
1 teaspoon salt

DIRECTIONS

Cook the chiles. Place the chiles, vinegar, and pineapple juice in a small saucepan, bring to a boil, and simmer, covered, for 12 minutes. Allow the liquid and chiles to cool.

Roast the garlic. Place the garlic in a small skillet over medium heat and cook, turning every so often, until it is a bit charred on the outside and very soft inside, 8–10 minutes. When the garlic is cool enough to handle, peel and roughly chop it.

Blend the salsa. Pour the chiles and their cooking liquid into a blender, add the garlic and salt, and blend to a purée, about 1 minute. Allow the sauce to cool and the acids to tone down the chile's heat for 2–3 hours before serving. Serve with Yucatecan dishes.

Arizona-style Salsa

About 1 cup. Nutrition information is for 1 tablespoon.

PER SERVING | 5 calories | 0 g protein
1 g carbohydrates | 0 g total fat
(0 g saturated) | 0 mg cholesterol
0 g fiber | 1 g sugar | 80 mg sodium

While less well known than Tex-Mex, Arizona has its own distinctive style of Mexican cooking that comes from the neighboring Mexican state of Sonora. The following is a favorite salsa that can be served with chips or antojitos.

INGREDIENTS

1 dried Anaheim (sometimes called California) chile, or a mild, dried New Mexico chile, toasted and rehydrated (pages 15–16)
3 chiles de árbol, toasted and rehydrated (pages 15–16)
1 (8–12 ounce) tomato, roasted (page 17)
½ tablespoon rice vinegar
½ teaspoon salt

DIRECTIONS

Make the salsa. Put all the ingredients in a blender and blend for 1–2 minutes, or until smooth.

Pasilla Chile Salsa

About 2 cups. Nutrition information is for 1 tablespoon.

PER SERVING | 0 calories | 0 g protein
1 g carbohydrates | 0 g total fat
(0 g saturated) | 0 mg cholesterol
0 g fiber | 1 g sugar | 55 mg sodium

I found this salsa at my favorite lobster restaurant in Puerto Nuevo, Baja California, a seaside village famous for its deep-fried lobster dish (page 205). The salsa also goes beautifully with smoked or grilled foods. Just be sure not to mistake the true pasilla for ancho chiles, as they are often called in California.

INGREDIENTS

3 cloves garlic, unpeeled
2 teaspoons extra-virgin olive oil, or cooking spray to coat the garlic
2 very large pasilla chiles, or 2½ medium to large ones, toasted and rehydrated (pages 15–16)
1 teaspoon canned chipotle chile, or to taste
1¼ pounds tomatoes (about 2 large or 3 medium, roasted; page 17)
¼ teaspoon dried leaf oregano
¾ teaspoon salt
⅔ cup minced white onion

DIRECTIONS

Preheat your oven to 350°F.

Roast the garlic. Brush or spray garlic with some of the olive oil, wrap in foil, and bake until soft, 35–40 minutes. Peel and reserve the garlic.

Blend the ingredients. Place the rehydrated pasilla chiles, the chipotle chile, one of the tomatoes, the oregano, garlic, and salt in the jar of a blender or in a food processor and blend to a smooth purée. Add the remaining tomato and pulse until it is combined with the other ingredients, but leave the salsa with some texture.

Finish the salsa. Put the remaining olive oil in a skillet over medium heat, add the onions, and sauté until they are just beginning to soften. Combine the onions with the rest of the salsa in a bowl.

Salsa X'nipek

DOG'S SNOUT SALSA

About 2 cups. Nutrition information is for 1 tablespoon.

PER SERVING | 5 calories | 0 g protein
1 g carbohydrates | 0 g total fat
(0 g saturated) | 0 mg cholesterol
0 g fiber | 1 g sugar | 30 mg sodium

Pronounced "shnee-PECK," this salsa from Yucatán state is made with fiery habanero chiles and the region's sour orange juice (or the suggested substitute). It is a refreshing version of the better known pico de gallo or salsa mexicana and goes especially well with Yucatán-style dishes, such as Pescado Pibil or Pollo Pibil. Do not be deceived by the small amount of chile; there's plenty! Allow the salsa to sit for at least an hour after making it to give the acid time to moderate the chile's heat and for the flavors to meld. The sauce does not keep well, so plan to use it the day it is made.

INGREDIENTS

1⅓ cups chopped tomatoes

⅔ cup finely chopped red onion

1 habanero chile, stemmed, seeded, veins removed,
    and very finely chopped

¼ cup finely chopped cilantro

4 tablespoons sour orange juice, or substitute 2 tablespoons
    freshly squeezed lime juice and 2 tablespoons freshly
    squeezed orange juice

¼ heaping teaspoon salt

DIRECTIONS

Make the salsa. Gently toss together everything except the salt. Allow the salsa to marinate, stirring it occasionally, for 1–2 hours at room temperature. Stir in the salt and serve. (The salt is not added initially because it will cause the tomatoes to become watery.)

Ancho and Chile de Árbol Salsa

About 2 cups. Nutrition information is for 1 tablespoon.

PER SERVING | 5 calories | 0 g protein
1 g carbohydrates | 0 g total fat
(0 g saturated) | 0 mg cholesterol
0 g fiber | 1 g sugar | 75 mg sodium

If I could have only one salsa, it might be this rustic one from Mexico's interior. It is terrific with just about anything, including broiled items, antojitos, and tortilla chips. In a pinch it can even be used as an enchilada sauce. It is also quite easy to prepare.

INGREDIENTS

½ pound tomatillos, husked and rinsed

4 chiles de árbol, toasted and rehydrated (pages 15–16)

1 ancho chile, toasted and rehydrated (pages 15–16),
    ⅓ cup of the soaking water reserved

1 tomato (about ½ pound), roasted (page 17)

1 teaspoon agave nectar or sugar

1 teaspoon salt

½ cup finely chopped white onion

DIRECTIONS

Cook the tomatillos. Put the tomatillos in a small saucepan, cover them with water, bring them to a boil, and simmer until they are soft but not falling apart, 3–5 minutes. Drain and reserve.

Finish the salsa. Put the chiles in a blender and add the reserved ⅓ cup of soaking water. Add the tomatillos, tomato, agave nectar, and salt to the blender and blend until completely puréed. Pour the salsa into a serving dish and stir in the onions.

Chile Pequín Salsa

Although this salsa is made with the fiery little chile pequín, because of its small size and rounded oblong shape, the final amount can be accurately measured and the piquancy controlled by using more or fewer chiles. Use the salsa in moderation to flavor steak, seafood, or pork.

About 1 cup. Nutrition information is for 1 tablespoon.

PER SERVING | 5 calories | 0 g protein
1 g carbohydrates | 0 g total fat
(0 g saturated) | 0 mg cholesterol
0 g fiber | 1 g sugar | 80 mg sodium

INGREDIENTS

1 large tomato (about 8 ounces)
½ cup chopped white onion
1 large or 2 small cloves garlic, minced
1 tablespoon chile pequín
½ teaspoon rice vinegar
⅛ teaspoon ground cloves
½ teaspoon salt

DIRECTIONS

Cook the vegetables. Bring enough water to cover the tomato to a boil and add the tomato, onion, and garlic. Simmer for 10 minutes, or until the tomato is quite soft.

Finish the salsa. Peel the tomato and discard the skin. Put the tomato, onion, and garlic in a food processor, add the remaining ingredients, and process until puréed. Allow about 15 minutes for the chiles to rehydrate, and process again before serving.

The Ultimate Mojo de Ajo Sauce

Mojo de ajo (garlic sauce) is served with seafood throughout Mexico. Usually, the garlic is simply fried in a little oil. I found this much more interesting version in a taquería in Saltillo, where it was served with tacos and on steak, as well as with seafood. While the salsa is high in calories, a little goes a long way, it is usually served with very low-calorie seafood, and it is made with healthy ingredients.

About ¾ cup. Nutrition information is for 1 tablespoon.

PER SERVING | 100 calories | 1 g protein
3 g carbohydrates | 9 g total fat
(1.5 g saturated) | 0 mg cholesterol
0 g fiber | 1 g sugar | 105 mg sodium

INGREDIENTS

3 chiles de árbol, seeded and coarsely chopped, or substitute a finely chopped canned chipotle chile
4 sun-dried tomatoes (not packed in oil), very finely chopped
¼ cup garlic chopped into ⅛-inch or slightly larger pieces
¼ cup minced white onion
½ teaspoon salt
½ cup extra-virgin olive oil
¼ heaping teaspoon freshly ground black pepper
1½ tablespoons dried cilantro
½ tablespoon freshly squeezed lime juice

Make the sauce. Place the chiles, tomatoes, garlic, onion, salt, oil, and pepper in a small saucepan over medium-low heat and cook until the oil just begins to bubble. Keep adjusting the heat so that the mixture cooks at the barest simmer, with just a few bubbles. Cook until the garlic is very soft and just beginning to brown, 30–45 minutes, stirring every 5 minutes or so. Add the cilantro and lime juice and simmer an additional 10 minutes, or until the garlic *just* begins to take on a golden hue (unless you prefer the stronger taste of browned garlic).

Salsa de Chile

CHILE SAUCE

About 2½ cups. Nutrition information is for 1 tablespoon and 1 cup.

PER SERVING | 10 calories | 0 g protein
1 g carbohydrates | 0 g total fat
(0 g saturated) | 0 mg cholesterol
0 g fiber | 0 g sugar | 45 mg sodium

PER 1-CUP SERVING | 150 calories
14 g protein | 16 g carbohydrates
16 g total fat (1 g saturated)
10 mg cholesterol | g fiber
1 g sugar | 1740 mg sodium

This is one of the most useful salsas. While it can be used as a salsa, it is even more functional as a sauce for anything from Chilaquiles (page 108) to the Santa Maria–style Beans (page 68). It is also very good as an enchilada sauce, especially when used to dip tortillas before wrapping them around a filling, as in the Interior-style Enchiladas (page 137). For that reason, the nutrition numbers are given for the salsa measurement of 1 tablespoon and for 1 cup. You can make it with New Mexico, guajillo, or ancho chiles in the portions listed in the recipe.

INGREDIENTS

8 mild to medium-hot New Mexico dried red chiles, 12 guajillo chiles, or 4 medium-sized ancho chiles, stemmed, seeded, toasted, and rehydrated (pages 15–16), 4 cups soaking water reserved
4 cloves garlic, chopped
1 teaspoon dried leaf oregano
1 tablespoon extra-virgin olive oil
1 teaspoon rice vinegar
2 bay leaves
¾ teaspoon salt, or to taste

DIRECTIONS

Blend the sauce ingredients. Put the chiles in a blender, add the garlic, oregano, and 2 cups of the reserved chile soaking water, and blend for 2 minutes, or until thoroughly puréed. Add the remaining 2 cups chile soaking water and blend another minute.

Cook the sauce. Heat a large saucepan over medium heat, add the olive oil, and stir in the blended sauce ingredients. Add the vinegar and bay leaves, bring to a boil, and cook at a medium simmer until the sauce is just thick enough to coat the back of a spoon, or the consistency of a very thin milkshake, 15–20 minutes. If the sauce thickens too much, add a little more water. If it is too thin, cook it a little longer. Add the salt and simmer another minute.

Cebollas en Escabeche

PICKLED ONIONS

About 2 cups. Nutrition information is for 2 tablespoons.

PER SERVING | 10 calories | 0 g protein
2 g carbohydrates | 0 g total fat
(0 g saturated) | 0 mg cholesterol
0 g fiber | 1 g sugar | 10 mg sodium

In Mexico's Yucatán state, pickled red onions are often used as a garnish or relish for everything from tacos to seafood, meats, and poultry. There are many recipes, some as simple as just marinating slightly blanched onions in lime juice. The following, which I adapted from one by Jacqueline Higuera McMahan, is by far my favorite, and it is very easy to prepare. It can be made picante by including the optional habanero chile. Nutrition calculations are based on 2 tablespoons rather than 1 tablespoon, as with most of the salsas.

INGREDIENTS

½ cup rice vinegar
¼ cup water
½ tablespoon extra-virgin olive oil
1 teaspoon dried leaf oregano
1 bay leaf
⅛ teaspoon salt
1 clove garlic, peeled and smashed
⅛ teaspoon whole dried thyme
1 small habanero chile, cut in half (optional)
1 (12-ounce) red onion, cut into ⅓-inch rings

DIRECTIONS

Make the onions. Put all the ingredients except the onion in a large saucepan and simmer for 3 minutes. Place the onions in a nonreactive bowl and pour the hot liquid over them. Let the onions sit at room temperature for 2 hours, stirring every half hour. Refrigerate.

Pico de Gallo, or Salsa Mexicana

About 2 cups. Nutrition information is for 1 tablespoon.

PER SERVING | 5 calories | 0 g protein
1 g carbohydrates | 0 g total fat
(0 g saturated) | 0 mg cholesterol
0 g fiber | 0 g sugar | 0 mg sodium

More of a relish than a salsa, in the United States Pico de Gallo has become a staple in Mexican American restaurants and is nearly always served with fajitas. In Mexico it is often referred to as Salsa Mexicana.

INGREDIENTS

1 cup finely chopped tomato
⅔ cup finely chopped white onion
2 tablespoons finely chopped serrano chiles
½ cup loosely packed minced cilantro

DIRECTIONS

Make the relish. Combine the ingredients.

Olive Salsa

About 1½ cups. Nutrition information is for 1 tablespoon.

PER SERVING | 20 calories | 0 g protein
2 g carbohydrates | 1 g total fat
(0 g saturated) | 0 mg cholesterol
0 g fiber | 0 g sugar | 55 mg sodium

This versatile salsa comes from Old Spanish California, where New World ingredients were adapted to traditional Spanish recipes. It is really two salsas in one recipe, depending on what kind of olives and peppers you decide to use. If using mild black California olives, I suggest the piquillo or red bell peppers, while the Anaheim chiles go wonderfully with manzanilla olives. As with some moles, the seeds of the chiles are toasted and ground to become a subtle but savory addition. Besides their use as a salsa on antojitos, these recipes work well to spice up bland items and are particularly good on baked potatoes and other vegetables, as well as on salads. They can also be combined with cheese, ham or other deli meats, or tuna to make delicious sandwiches and are tasty over sliced hard-boiled eggs.

INGREDIENTS

3 mild dried New Mexico red chiles
½ cup very finely chopped white onion
¾ cup very finely chopped mild black California pitted olives or green manzanilla olives
½ cup roasted, peeled, very finely chopped piquillo chile, red bell pepper, or roasted and peeled Anaheim chiles
2 green onions, very finely chopped
½ teaspoon dried leaf oregano
1 teaspoon agave nectar, or substitute honey
¼ teaspoon salt
¼ teaspoon finely ground black pepper
1 tablespoon extra-virgin olive oil
¼ cup plus 2 tablespoons rice vinegar

DIRECTIONS

Preheat your oven to 275°F.

Dry and crush the chiles. Bake the New Mexico chiles on a small baking sheet until they are well toasted but not burned, about 10 minutes. They should still be a bit soft but will quickly become dry and brittle. If they do not turn brittle, heat them a little longer. Tear open the chiles, put the seeds into a small dish, and reserve. Pulse the chiles in a food processor until they are the consistency of very fine chile flakes. You can also chop the chiles by hand, but that can be both tedious and messy. Put the flakes in another bowl and reserve.

Toast and grind the chile seeds. Toast the seeds in a small dry skillet over medium heat until golden brown. Grind them to a powder in a spice or coffee grinder and add them to the chile flakes.

Finish the salsa. Stir in the remaining ingredients and refrigerate for at least 2 hours before serving to allow the flavors to meld.

Salsa de Molcajete

About 1 cup. Nutrition information is for 1 tablespoon.

PER SERVING | 10 calories | 0 g protein
1 g carbohydrates | 0 g total fat
(0 g saturated) | 0 mg cholesterol
0 g fiber | 0 g sugar | 110 mg sodium

Salsa de Molcajete is a tradition at some Mexico City restaurants and cantinas, and there is no more authentic salsa. The preparation is great fun at home, especially when you have guests, and it is a perfect vehicle for individual or collective creativity. Here's how it went at a famous cantina. A chef brought an array of tempting ingredients and a molcajete to our table. After an initial consultation, he added and ground ingredients one at a time. The molcajete slowly filled, emitting the intoxicating aroma of its alluring ingredients.

Commonly used items include salt; garlic; chopped onion; toasted sesame seeds (heat them in an ungreased skillet over medium heat, stirring often until they are golden brown); a selection of dried chiles, such as ancho, pasilla, pequín (break the larger chiles into small pieces and cook them over medium heat in just enough oil to film the surface of a skillet until they begin to crisp [but not burn], then chop them finely before adding them to the molcajete); fresh chiles, such as serranos, jalapeños, and poblanos (all of which should be roasted or boiled and cut into manageable pieces); canned chipotle chiles and/or their adobo sauce; tomatoes (roasted until their skins can be removed and they are very soft); husked tomatillos (roasted, but they do not need to be peeled); cilantro; limes for juice; dried oregano; and mint.

Adding a little salt to the molcajete will help reduce the ingredients to a coarse texture and will make grinding harder items such as garlic and onions much easier. Add a little water to thin the salsa toward the end. If you cannot find a molcajete, a rough-surfaced Oriental mortar and pestle will work. Make sure everything to be added to the molcajete can be easily ground. Dried chiles should first be fried in just a little oil until they are crisp enough to grind easily, but care must be taken not to overcook them, which will make them bitter. They should be chopped into small pieces before adding them to the molcajete. Fresh chiles and tomatoes should be roasted or broiled to make them soft and to facilitate removing their skins.

If you wish, begin by following the recipe below.

INGREDIENTS

¾ teaspoon salt

2 cloves garlic

2 tablespoons finely chopped white onion

2 teaspoons toasted sesame seeds

1 small jalapeño chile, roasted and peeled (page 16)

1 chile de árbol, toasted in an oil-filmed skillet until crisp but not burned

1 very small pasilla chile, toasted in an oil-filmed skillet until crisp but not burned

⅔ of 1 small ancho chile, toasted in an oil-filmed skillet until crisp but not burned

2 chiles pequín, toasted in an oil-filmed skillet until crisp
but not burned
1 tomato, broiled and peeled (page 17)
Water as needed to get the consistency you want

DIRECTIONS

Make the salsa. Add the salt to the *molcajete*. Add the ingredients one at a time, grinding each one to the texture you want before adding the next.

Yucatán-style Tomato Salsa

About 1¼ cups. Nutrition information is for 1 tablespoon.

PER SERVING | 15 calories | 0 g protein
1 g carbohydrates | 1 g total fat
(0 g saturated) | 0 mg cholesterol
0 g fiber | 1 g sugar | 20 mg sodium

This salsa uses fiery habanero chiles, but their heat is toned down to a subtle piquancy by cooking them halved rather than chopped and removing them when the salsa is finished. Use it like any salsa and in the preparation of the area's delicious Huevos Motuleños (page 104) and Papadzules (page 222).

INGREDIENTS

2½ cups water
1 pound (about 2 medium-sized) tomatoes
1 habanero chile, cut in half
1½ tablespoons extra-virgin olive oil
½ cup chopped white onion
⅛ heaping teaspoon salt

DIRECTIONS

Cook the tomatoes. Bring the water to a boil and add the tomatoes and chiles. Simmer for 4 minutes, or until the tomatoes are beginning to soften. Remove the tomatoes and chiles from the pan; allow the tomatoes to cool slightly then remove and discard their skins and put the tomatoes in a food processor fitted with the steel blade. Reserve the cooking liquid if you plan to make Papadzules or need to thin the sauce. Reserve the chiles separately.

Cook the onions and purée the sauce. Heat a skillet over medium heat, add ½ tablespoon of the oil and the onions, and sauté, stirring frequently, until the onions just begin to turn golden. Put the onions in the food processor with the tomatoes and process for 1 minute. Put the sauce through a strainer or food mill to remove the seeds.

Cook the tomato sauce. Heat a small saucepan over medium heat, add the remaining tablespoon oil, the sauce, and the salt. If you think the sauce needs more heat, add back the habanero halves. Bring the sauce to a boil and simmer until it is thick enough to hold its shape, 2–5 minutes. Thin with reserved liquid if you like a thinner sauce. If you used the chiles, remove and discard them.

Romesco Sauce

About 1 cup. Nutrition information is for 1 tablespoon.

PER SERVING | 50 calories | 0 g protein
1 g carbohydrates | 5 g total fat
(0.5 g saturated) | 0 mg cholesterol
0 g fiber | 1 g sugar | 115 mg sodium

Made primarily with what some nutritionists call superfoods, this is one of the healthiest sauces there are when used in small quantities. It is also one of my favorites, in addition to Chimichurri Sauce (page 51), to serve with grilled foods, and it is a snap to prepare. In Spain, Romesco Sauce has many variations, sometimes including roasted red peppers, olives, tomatoes, and bread crumbs. This simple version uses Mexico's smoked chipotle chiles and Spain's incomparable smoked paprika. The recipe makes a terrific substitute for béarnaise and hollandaise sauces, mayonnaise dressings, tartar sauce, and aioli, and it complements seafood, beef, poultry, vegetables, and eggs.

INGREDIENTS

1 cup cherry tomatoes
2 tablespoons roasted and skinned whole almonds
3 garlic cloves, peeled and cut in half lengthwise
1 small to medium canned chipotle chile, seeded and chopped
½ heaping teaspoon salt
1 tablespoon sherry vinegar (or freshly squeezed lime or lemon juice for use with seafood)
⅓ cup extra-virgin olive oil
½ teaspoon sweet smoked Spanish paprika
2 tablespoons minced parsley

DIRECTIONS

Dry roast the tomatoes, nuts, and garlic. Heat an ungreased skillet over medium-high to high heat until it is very hot. Place the tomatoes, almonds, and garlic in the skillet and cook, stirring almost constantly, until the tomatoes are blackened and *just* starting to deflate. Don't worry if the nuts and garlic appear burned; that just enhances the flavor. Do make sure that the garlic is cooked through.

Finish the sauce. Place the tomatoes, almonds, and garlic in a food processor, add the remaining ingredients, and process in pulses until the sauce is thick but still has some texture.

Chimichurri Sauce

About ¾ cup. Nutrition information is for 1 tablespoon.

PER SERVING | 90 calories | 0 g protein
2 g carbohydrates | 9 g total fat
(1.5 g saturated) | 0 mg cholesterol
0 g fiber | 1 g sugar | 125 mg sodium

While this sauce is of Argentine rather than Mexican origin, I have had it in one version or another many times in Mexico—probably because it is such a perfect accompaniment to broiled meats, poultry, and seafood. When it is served with the Romesco Sauce, diners have a wonderful choice between bold and rustic flavors. I have tried many versions of Chimichurri Sauce, and this one is my favorite. Please note that while the recipe calls for chile flakes, the best choice is Aleppo chile flakes. Grown in Syria and Turkey, they are a bit like ancho chiles, but a little hotter. They are also crushed without the seeds, which avoids the unpleasant bitterness and texture of most other kinds. They are available from Penzey's Spices. While the sauce is made mostly with high-calorie olive oil, like its cousin, the Ultimate Mojo de Ajo Sauce, a little goes a very long way, and it makes whatever it is served with a real reward.

INGREDIENTS

½ cup extra-virgin olive oil
6 cloves garlic, very finely chopped or put through a garlic press
1 tablespoon dried leaf oregano
2 teaspoons chile flakes
4 teaspoons red wine vinegar
½ teaspoon salt
¼ teaspoon freshly ground black pepper
¼ cup finely chopped parsley

DIRECTIONS

Heat the garlic and spices. Put the olive oil, garlic, oregano, and chile flakes into a small microwave-safe dish and microwave to about 135°–150°F on an instant-read thermometer, about 30 seconds on High. You want to heat the garlic just enough to release its flavor, but not so much that it actually cooks or makes the oil turn cloudy. Allow the oil to cool to room temperature.

Finish the sauce. Stir in the vinegar, salt, pepper, and parsley and allow the flavors to meld for an hour or 2 before serving.

Cranberry-Jalapeño Jelly

1–1¼ cups. Nutrition information is for 1 tablespoon.

PER SERVING | 35 calories | 0 g protein
8 g carbohydrates | 0 g total fat
(0 g saturated) | 0 mg cholesterol
0 g fiber | 8 g sugar | 20 mg sodium

I don't remember where I found this recipe or if I was the one who added the jalapeño to it. In any case, in addition to being far superior to commercial cranberry sauces, it is also simple and fun to prepare. It goes particularly well with poultry and pork, and I always serve a tablespoon or two of it with the Grilled Quail (page 165). If you want more or less heat, just add more or less jalapeño.

INGREDIENTS

½ cup water
½ cup sugar
1 cup fresh cranberries
¼ cup finely chopped dried apricots
Pinch of salt
1 small jalapeño, stems and seeds removed, very finely chopped
Grated zest from ½ orange

DIRECTIONS

Make the syrup. Cook the water and sugar at a low to medium boil for 5 minutes.

Finish the jelly. Add the cranberries, apricots, salt, and jalapeño and cook them at a low to medium simmer for 6 minutes, at which time the cranberries should be breaking apart. Add the orange zest and continue to simmer, stirring, until thick, about 1 minute.

BOTANAS

APPETIZERS

THIS SECTION contains recipes for foods that are usually served just as appetizers or snacks. Many other recipes (a partial list appears below) can be easily adapted for use as *botanas* by serving them in smaller portions:

- ▸ Huitlacoche-stuffed Mushrooms (page 223)
- ▸ Shrimp Salad (page 98)
- ▸ Smoked Salmon Tacos, made with small tortillas (page 128)
- ▸ Mushroom Quesadillas, cut in half or made with small tortillas (page 145)
- ▸ Spinach Quesadillas, cut in half or made with small tortillas (page 146)
- ▸ Huitlacoche and Mushroom Quesadillas, cut in half or made with small tortillas (page 146)

Tuna Ceviche

6 appetizer servings,
4 as an entrée

PER SERVING | 130 calories
19 g protein | 10 g carbohydrates
1.5 g total fat (0 g saturated)
30 mg cholesterol | 1 g fiber
7 g sugar | 135 mg sodium

This delicious and relatively quick ceviche was adapted from one served by Chef Miguel Ravago at the terrific Fonda San Miguel restaurant in Austin, Texas. Many supermarkets now carry frozen yellowfin or ahi tuna that is labeled "sashimi quality." That means it is safe to eat raw, and that is what you should use. Other than a bit of slicing and juicing, this recipe could not be easier or tastier, but it will be no better than the juices you use, so they should be freshly squeezed. I often serve this for a light supper with a half avocado on the side.

INGREDIENTS

For the ceviche dressing

1 cup matchstick-size pieces of red onion, about 1 inch long and
    less than ⅛-inch thick
2 tablespoons matchstick-size pieces of peeled gingerroot,
    about 1 inch long and no thicker than a toothpick
2 tablespoons seeded serrano chile, cut same size as gingerroot
½ cup freshly squeezed lime juice
½ cup freshly squeezed orange juice
½ cup freshly squeezed grapefruit juice
1 teaspoon agave nectar or sugar
1 teaspoon sea salt
2 tablespoons extra-virgin olive oil

To finish

1 cup sliced red bell pepper, ⅛-inch thick and 1 inch long
1 cup sliced mango, ⅛-inch thick by about 1 inch in length and width
1 pound yellowfin (ahi) tuna, cut into ½-inch pieces
¼ cup loosely packed chopped cilantro

DIRECTIONS

Make the dressing. To remove any off flavors, soak the onion, gingerroot, and serrano chile for a few minutes in ice-cold water. While they are soaking, combine the juices, agave nectar, salt, and olive oil. Drain and pat dry the onion, gingerroot, and serrano, add to the dressing, and refrigerate for 1 hour for the flavors to meld.

Finish the ceviche. Stir in the bell pepper, mango, tuna, and cilantro and refrigerate for 15 minutes before serving.

Vuelva a la Vida

RETURN TO LIFE

4 servings

PER SERVING | 210 calories
18 g protein | 24 g carbohydrates
4.5 g total fat (0.5 g saturated)
145 mg cholesterol | 1 g fiber
9 g sugar | 300 mg sodium

This seafood cocktail is also a traditional hangover remedy in Mexico. It makes a great appetizer or light lunch and can be prepared with any combination of seafood, including fish, shrimp, scallops, crab, and octopus. If you are in a hurry, use precooked shrimp and crabmeat. In Mexico it is often served with saltine crackers, which come in a low-sodium version.

INGREDIENTS

⅓ cup low-salt catsup
⅓ cup freshly squeezed orange juice
¼ cup tomato juice
1 teaspoon minced, canned chipotle chile
1 teaspoon adobo from the can of chipotle chiles
2 tablespoons minced onion, rinsed with cold water and dried
½ cup finely chopped fresh tomato
1 tablespoon minced cilantro
½ tablespoon minced parsley
¼ teaspoon dried leaf oregano
½ tablespoon extra-virgin olive oil
2 tablespoons freshly squeezed lime juice
1 pound boiled and chilled shrimp (weighed after peeling), crab, fish, or a combination, refrigerated
20 low-salt saltine crackers

DIRECTIONS

Whisk everything together except the seafood and crackers and chill. This can be done several days ahead of serving. Stir the chilled seafood into the sauce and serve with the saltines.

Pickled Chiles and Vegetables

About 16 appetizer servings

PER SERVING | 30 calories | 0 g protein
4 g carbohydrates | 1.5 g total fat
(0 g saturated) | 0 mg cholesterol
1 g fiber | 2 g sugar | 125 mg sodium

For years I enjoyed the pickled chiles, carrots, and other vegetables served as an appetizer in Mexican restaurants, mostly south of the border. I tried several recipes that were decent, but I always felt they could be better. Then I tried them at the La Canasta restaurant in Saltillo, and they were the best I'd ever had. I raved about them to such an extent that the owners graciously gave me the recipe. The following is my adaptation. Usually, ingredients are cooked in a combination of vinegar, water, herbs, and a little oil. In this recipe, the chiles are cured overnight rather than cooked. Except for the carrots, the other ingredients are given only brief dips in boiling water.

INGREDIENTS

½ cup water

2¼ teaspoons salt

¼ cup plus 2 tablespoons rice vinegar

1 tablespoon freshly squeezed lime juice

4 ounces jalapeño peppers, stems and seeds removed, cut into strips about ½-inch wide and 2½ inches long (weighed after being stemmed and seeded)

3 cloves garlic, peeled and smashed

¼ cup plus 2 tablespoons corn oil, plus a little extra for cooking the garlic

¼ heaping teaspoon dried leaf oregano

¼ heaping teaspoon dried thyme

¼ heaping teaspoon dried marjoram

¼ teaspoon finely ground black pepper

3 bay leaves

8 ounces carrots, peeled and cut into strips about 2½ inches long by ½-inch wide and ¼-inch thick

4 ounces white onion, peeled and cut into strips about 2½ inches long by ½-inch wide

6 ounces zucchini or yellow squash, or a combination, cut into strips about 2½ inches long by ½ inch wide and ¼ inch thick

3 ounces jícama, peeled and cut into pieces about $\frac{1}{16}$-inch thick and 1 inch in diameter

DIRECTIONS

Make the first-stage pickling liquid. The night before serving, dissolve the salt in the water in a nonreactive bowl. Add the vinegar and lime juice and mix well.

Prep and add the jalapeños. Prick the jalapeños all over with a fork or, much easier, use a spring-loaded meat tenderizer. Put the jalapeños in the pickling liquid and refrigerate overnight.

Cook and add the garlic. Put the garlic in a very small microwave-safe bowl and barely cover it with oil. Microwave on High until the garlic is soft, about 35 seconds. Discard the oil and stir the garlic into the jalapeños.

Finish the pickling liquid. Add the ¼ cup plus 2 tablespoons corn oil to the pickling liquid and stir in the oregano, thyme, marjoram, pepper, and bay leaves.

Parboil the vegetables. Bring a large pot of water to a boil, add the carrots, and simmer until they *just* start to become tender. Put the carrots into ice water to stop the cooking. Using a large strainer, submerge the onions in the boiling water for 5 seconds then put them into ice water to stop the cooking. Submerge the squash in the boiling water for 15 seconds then put it into the ice water.

Complete the recipe. When the vegetables are cold, remove them from the ice water, pat them dry, and add them to the pickling liquid. Add the jícama and mix everything thoroughly. Refrigerate the vegetables for at least 3 hours, stirring every half hour. At first it will seem that there is not enough liquid, but with an occasional stirring, there will be. The vegetables will keep for at least a week refrigerated.

Hot Garlic Peanuts

12–16 appetizer servings of about 2 tablespoons each

PER SERVING | 130 calories | 6 g protein
4 g carbohydrates | 11 g total fat
(1.5 g saturated) | 0 mg cholesterol
2 g fiber | 0 g sugar | 50 mg sodium

Chile-spiced peanuts are a favorite snack in Mexico. Although they are high in calories, in small portions they are a delicious alternative to other snacks (that is, if you or your guests are not allergic to them). This is my version of the wonderful treats that used to be made by an old man in the border town of Piedras Negras. Sea salt is specified because in this application its pure flavor improves the dish. Be sure to use raw peanuts, meaning they have not been roasted or blanched. After roasting and cooling, the peanuts should be refrigerated and will keep at least a week.

INGREDIENTS

¼ cup dried pequín chiles

½ teaspoon dried leaf oregano

10 cloves garlic, separated into groups of 2 and 8, and then peeled and chopped into approximately ⅛-inch pieces

½ cup canola oil

12 ounces (about 2 cups) raw Spanish peanuts

¼ heaping teaspoon sea salt, or to taste ▸▸

Make the chile oil. Put the chiles, oregano, and 2 of the chopped garlic cloves in a small saucepan. Add the oil and turn the heat to medium. As soon as you see more than a few bubbles rise from the bottom of the pan (if you have an instant-read thermometer, that will be about when the temperature reaches 205°F), remove the pan from the heat. Do not allow the oil to reach a full simmer. Pour the warm oil and chiles into a blender and blend for 2 minutes. Leave in the blender for 20 minutes. Blend again then push the contents through a fine strainer lined with cheesecloth. You should have about ¼ cup chile oil with very little sediment.

Preheat your oven to 350°F.

Make the peanuts. Put the peanuts into a 9-inch iron skillet or a ridged baking sheet large enough to hold them in a single layer. Toss the peanuts with 1 tablespoon of the chile oil and put them in the oven. Bake for 10 minutes. Stir and bake for 10 more minutes. Stir in the remaining 8 chopped garlic cloves and cook for another 7 minutes. Remove the peanuts from the oven and immediately stir in the salt. At this point the nuts will still be a bit raw. Let them cool in the pan they were cooked in for 45 minutes, by which time they should be crunchy and delicious.

Pepitas

TOASTED PUMPKIN SEEDS

About 6 servings of 2 heaping tablespoons each

PER SERVING | 90 calories | 4 g protein
2 g carbohydrates | 7 g total fat
(1.5 g saturated) | 0 mg cholesterol
1 g fiber | 0 g sugar | 50 mg sodium

This popular appetizer and bar snack is made with one of the only plant foods that contain sizable amounts of healthy omega-3 fatty acids. The pumpkin seeds are "popped" in much the same way as popcorn. When I intend to use them as part of another recipe, I toast them without oil. When I make them for a snack or appetizer, I use just a little oil, which gives them a better mouthfeel and helps the seasonings adhere. If the seeds are not fresh, they will not pop properly, but they should still taste all right, just not as light and crunchy.

INGREDIENTS

¼ teaspoon extra-virgin olive oil
¾ cup hulled raw green pumpkin seeds
¼ teaspoon pure ancho or New Mexico chile powder
⅛ heaping teaspoon sea salt

DIRECTIONS

Preheat your oven to 425°F.

Put the pumpkin seeds in a 9-inch oven-safe skillet. I use an iron one or a similar-sized baking dish. Add the remaining ingredients and toss them with the seeds. Bake for 9–10 minutes. They are ready when they have popped. Do not let them scorch or they will be bitter.

Guacamole

*4 appetizer servings with chips or
as a garnish for antojitos*

PER SERVING | 80 calories | 1 g protein
5 g carbohydrates | 7 g total fat
(1 g saturated) | 0 mg cholesterol
3 g fiber | 1 g sugar | 180 mg sodium

So versatile is guacamole that it is always difficult to decide whether it is an appetizer, a salad, or a sauce. Whatever you call it, it is best made with Hass avocados or a similar variety—anything but the large, watery, smooth-skinned ones. Growers have learned how to peel, preserve, and package avocados, but to me they have an artificial flavor and lack the buttery goodness of a perfectly ripe avocado, so I use them only when fresh ones are unavailable.

To speed up the ripening process, put an unripe avocado in a plastic bag with 2 or 3 bananas. Please note that in the fall even the best avocado varieties lose some of their rich flavor for a month or two. Mexican chefs often compensate by adding about 1 tablespoon crema mexicana or sour cream. The following recipe, using 1 large avocado, makes a nice appetizer dip or topping for tacos for 4 people.

INGREDIENTS

1 large avocado (6–7 ounces after peeling and seeding)
¼ heaping teaspoon kosher salt, or to taste
2 teaspoons freshly squeezed lime juice, or to taste
3 tablespoons finely chopped onion, rinsed in cold water and drained
1–2 tablespoons finely chopped stemmed and seeded serrano chile
3 tablespoons finely chopped Roma tomato
2 tablespoons finely chopped cilantro

DIRECTIONS

With a sharp knife, cut the avocado in half lengthwise down to the seed. Move the knife in a circle around the fruit to cut the avocado in half. Twist the halves apart, remove the seed, and with a spoon scoop the flesh into a *molcajete* or large mortar and pestle and chop it into large pieces. Add the salt and lime juice to the avocado and mash to the desired texture (I like it a little chunky). Add the remaining ingredients and mix with a spoon.

RICE, BEANS

& OTHER SIDE DISHES

RICE

Besides different varieties, rice comes in two basic forms, brown and white. When processing brown rice, only the outer husk is removed. To make white rice, the outer husk is stripped off and then the bran and germ layers are also removed. This process eliminates vitamins and minerals such as B_1, B_3, iron, and magnesium. Some but not all of these may be "added back," but there are questions regarding the effectiveness of the enrichment process. Additionally, it is believed that the oil in rice bran may help lower LDL, or bad cholesterol.

For these reasons, nutrition experts tell us that we should eat brown rather than white rice. There are two problems with this. First, brown rice usually turns out more like a gloppy, unappetizing mess than the light, steamed grains we want. Second, even if we do make it properly, for many used to white rice, brown rice simply does not taste right. The brown rice recipe I present here (page 64), adapted from one that appeared in the April/May 2005 issue of *Fine Cooking* magazine, definitely solves the first problem. While there may be no solution for the second one that suits everyone, what works well for me is to combine cooked brown and white rice on a half-and-half basis. I suggest you try that, varying the proportions to suit your taste.

Although in Mexico medium-grain rice is often used, I prefer long-grain, and my favorite is aromatic jasmine. Most Mexican rice is cooked pilaf-style, which means the rice is fried before being steamed. Mexican rice often needs to be soaked and rinsed to remove the starch before it is cooked. However, when prepared pilaf-style, rice from U.S. supermarkets usually does not require this step.

Most Mexican cooks add things like onion, garlic, and oregano to both rice and bean recipes. However, I have found that also blending some of those important flavors into the water or broth in which the rice and beans are cooked, and which they absorb in the process, produces a more savory result.

Please note that all the pilaf-style rice heats up well in a microwave, so it can be prepared even several days ahead of serving.

Arroz a la Mexicana

MEXICAN RICE

~~~~~~~~~~~~~~~~~~

8 servings

PER SERVING | 220 calories | 4 g protein
33 g carbohydrates | 7 g total fat
(1 g saturated) | 0 mg cholesterol
2 g fiber | 3 g sugar | 350 mg sodium

This is one of the world's greatest rice dishes—but only when it is prepared properly, which is seldom. What makes it so special is that, like all pilaf-style rice, it is first fried in oil, which keeps the grains from sticking together and gives the rice a toasty flavor and texture. It is then fried in a tomato sauce until the liquid has evaporated; this cooks the flavor into the rice without making it gloppy. The rice is finished in a savory broth, which instills yet another layer of flavor. Because the process is a bit difficult in very large quantities, many restaurants take shortcuts, but that is not necessary at home.

INGREDIENTS

2 cloves garlic, chopped

1 teaspoon salt

2⅓ cups low-sodium chicken broth

¼ cup extra-virgin olive oil

1½ cups long-grain rice, preferably jasmine

⅓ cup canned, fire-roasted crushed tomatoes, or substitute tomato sauce

⅓ cup peeled and grated carrot

1 cup sliced white onion, ¼-inch thick

1 cup sliced, seeded poblano chile, ¼-inch thick

¼ cup frozen peas

DIRECTIONS

Prepare the broth. Put the garlic and the salt in a blender, add 1 cup of the broth, and purée. Add the rest of the broth and blend again to mix thoroughly. Reserve.

Fry the rice. Heat a large pot (I like to use a cast iron Dutch oven) over medium heat, add the olive oil, and stir in the rice. Cook the rice, stirring frequently, until it turns golden brown. If necessary, turn the heat down to keep it from scorching. When it is done, in 5–8 minutes, you will hear a sound like sand being tossed in a metal container.

Cook the sauce into the rice. Stir the crushed tomato or tomato sauce into the browned rice, turn the heat to medium or just a bit over, and cook, stirring almost constantly, until nearly all the liquid has evaporated and the rice grains no longer stick together, about 5 minutes. This is very important, as the more liquid that has evaporated the lighter the rice will be. At first you will think it's never going to happen, but it will. Toward the end, some of the rice may begin to scorch. A little of that adds to the flavor, but lower the heat to minimize it. ▶▶

Cook the rice. Blend the broth mixture briefly and pour it into the pot with the rice. Raise the heat to high and add the carrots, sliced onion, poblano, and frozen peas. Bring the broth to a full boil, cover the pot, turn the heat as low as you can to keep the broth at a simmer, and cook for 15 minutes. Remove the pot from the heat and let the rice steam for 10 minutes. Remove the lid and gently stir the rice with a fork to separate the grains. Cover the pot and allow the rice to steam for 10 more minutes.

Saffron Rice

8–10 servings

PER SERVING | 190 calories | 3 g protein 28 g carbohydrates | 6 g total fat (2.5 g saturated) | 10 mg cholesterol 0 g fiber | 0 g sugar | 320 mg sodium

The elegant taste of saffron brings Mexico's Spanish heritage to the table with this terrific rice dish. Like other pilaf-style rice, it can be made a day or two in advance and successfully reheated in a microwave.

INGREDIENTS

1 pinch (about ¼ packed teaspoon) saffron threads
3 cups low-sodium chicken broth
4 cloves garlic, minced
1 teaspoon salt
½ tablespoon freshly squeezed lime juice
2 tablespoons extra-virgin olive oil
2 tablespoons butter substitute
1½ cups jasmine rice, or substitute any good long-grain rice
¼ cup minced white onion
1 medium serrano chile, seeds and veins removed and minced
2 tablespoons finely chopped parsley

DIRECTIONS

Infuse the broth with saffron. Place the saffron in a heat-proof bowl. Bring 1 cup of broth just to a boil and pour it over the saffron. Steep the mixture for at least 15 minutes.

Make the rest of the cooking liquid. Place 3 of the minced garlic cloves and the salt in a blender, add the remaining 2 cups broth and lime juice, and blend until puréed.

Cook the rice in the oil and butter. Heat a heavy pot over medium heat and add the olive oil and butter substitute. When the butter has melted, stir in the rice and cook for 3–5 minutes, stirring frequently, until it *just* begins to brown. Add the remaining minced clove of garlic, the onion, and chile to the rice and stir for 1 minute. Stir in the blended broth mixture and the saffron-infused broth and bring to a boil. Cover the pot, turn the heat as low as possible while keeping the liquid at a medium simmer, and cook the rice for 15 minutes.

Finish the rice. Remove the pot from the heat and allow the rice to steam, covered, for 10 minutes. Remove the lid and carefully stir the rice with a fork to separate the grains. Stir in the parsley, replace the lid, and allow the rice to sit for another 10 minutes before serving.

Arroz Huérfano

ORPHAN'S RICE

8–10 servings

PER SERVING | 340 calories
9 g protein | 32 g carbohydrates
21 g total fat (3.5 g saturated)
10 mg cholesterol | 2 g fiber
1 g sugar | 410 mg sodium

"Rich person's rice" would be a more appropriate name for this delicious dish, which takes the elegant Saffron Rice and kicks it up a notch. While this recipe has quite a few calories for a side dish, it can be served in much smaller portions, and friends in Mexico often serve it with a small salad or just sliced avocado to make an entire meal because the rice has a nice amount of protein.

INGREDIENTS

1 recipe Saffron Rice (page 62) prepared through the first 10 minutes
    of steaming, after the pot has been removed from the heat
1 tablespoon butter substitute
½ cup blanched slivered almonds
⅓ cup pecan halves
⅓ cup walnut halves
⅓ cup pine nuts
3 ounces lower-sodium ham, finely chopped

DIRECTIONS

Sauté the nuts. While the Saffron Rice is cooking, heat a skillet over medium heat. Add the butter substitute, and when it has melted, add the nuts. Sauté the nuts, stirring constantly, until the almonds begin to turn golden. Remove the skillet from the heat, stir in the ham, and set aside.

Finish the rice. After adding the parsley to the Saffron Rice, stir in the cooked nuts and ham, cover the pot, and allow the rice to steam for the final 10 minutes.

Brown Rice

5–7 half-cup servings

PER SERVING | 110 calories | 2 g protein
24 g carbohydrates | 1 g total fat
(0 g saturated) | 0 mg cholesterol
1 g fiber | 0 g sugar | 200 mg sodium

Brown rice can be eaten by itself or added to white rice to produce a healthier outcome with a nice nutty flavor. This is the best way I have found to prepare it.

INGREDIENTS

1 cup brown rice
6 cups water, plus water for rinsing
1½ teaspoons salt

DIRECTIONS

Rinse the rice. Place the rice in a bowl, cover it with water, and massage it for about 10 seconds. Place the rice in a strainer and rinse under cold running water for 15 seconds.

Cook the rice. In a large pot, bring the 6 cups of water and the salt to a boil. Add the rice and simmer, uncovered, for 30 minutes. Pour the rice into your strainer and allow it to drain for 15 seconds, discarding all the cooking water.

Steam the rice. Return the rice to the pot and cover it tightly. To make a good seal, sandwich a towel between the lid and the pot. Allow the rice to steam for 15 minutes off the heat. Stir the rice with a fork and serve or mix it with another rice.

BEANS

For centuries the Mexican diet was based on the staples of corn, beans, squash, and chiles, often grown together in small garden plots called *milpas*. Much of the nutritional benefit, including most of the protein, came from beans, and that is true to this day. A recent study concluded that a daily cup of beans, accompanied by one less sugary soda, could positively affect the incidence of diabetes in children.

Since I first began cooking, I have been told never to salt beans until the end of the cooking process, because doing so would make them tough. I followed this advice and have been pleased with the results. However, when I saw a recipe by the innovative folks at *Cook's Illustrated* that advised exactly the opposite, I could not resist trying it. They said to bring the beans to a boil with salted water, then cover and remove them from the heat and allow them to sit for

an hour. The results were tender, creamy, and delicious, some of the best beans I had ever had. After several more experiments with the same results, I decided to use that process for most of the following recipes.

Frijoles de Olla

POT BEANS

About 12 half-cup servings

PER SERVING | 100 calories | 6 g protein
18 g carbohydrates | 0 g total fat
(0 g saturated) | 0 mg cholesterol
4 g fiber | 1 g sugar | 220 mg sodium

Frijoles de Olla is the basic bean recipe from which more elaborate versions, such as Frijoles Borrachos and Frijoles a la Charra, are made. It is also the first step in making Frijoles Refritos (refried beans). The recipe works for most beans, including the most popular ones: pinto, black, pink, bayo, and peruano (Peruvian). Most cooks add the flavorings to the pot with the beans, but I have found that, as with rice, blending them with the cooking liquid, which is then absorbed into the beans, provides a more flavorful result. As mentioned in the introduction, I am using the cooking method which heats the beans in salted water and allows them to soak for one hour before finishing them. That process leaves the total cooking time about the same or perhaps adds an additional 15 minutes, but it produces delicious results.

Please note that when beans are cooked at a vigorous simmer, the skins will tend to come off and thicken the broth. Some cooks like this effect, while others prefer the beans to be more intact, with a thinner broth.

INGREDIENTS

4 quarts water
3 tablespoons salt
1 pound pinto or black beans, or any others mentioned above,
    picked over to remove any stones or broken beans
3 cloves garlic, chopped
⅓ cup chopped white onions
1 teaspoon dried leaf oregano
1 quart water, plus a little more, if needed
2 sprigs epazote (optional with black beans)
Salt to taste

DIRECTIONS

Heat and soak the beans. Put the 4 quarts water, salt, and beans into a pot (6 quarts is a good size). Bring to a full boil, cover the pot, remove it from the heat, and allow the beans to sit for 1 hour. Discard the soaking water, rinse the beans thoroughly, rinse out the pot, and return the beans to it.

Finish the beans. Put the garlic, onion, oregano, and 1 cup of the water in a blender and purée. Add 3 more cups water and blend briefly.

Pour the blended liquid into the pot with the beans, bring to a boil, and add the epazote, if using. Simmer the beans, covered except for about ½ inch, or just enough to allow some steam to escape, until they are tender. Depending on your altitude and how dry the beans were to begin with, this usually takes about a half hour. If it takes a little longer or if you cooked the beans at a rapid simmer, you may have to add a little more water to keep the beans covered. Remove the epazote and add salt to taste. I usually add none, and that is how the nutrition calculations were made. ▶▶

(To estimate the amount of sodium, I calculated the percentage of the liquid the beans absorbed during the soaking and assumed they absorbed salt in the same ratio.)

The beans are now ready to serve, for additional ingredients to be added to make more elaborate bean dishes, or to be made into refried beans.

Frijoles Charros or Borrachos

CHARRO OR DRUNKEN BEANS

About 7 cups, or 14 half-cup servings

PER SERVING | 150 calories | 8 g protein 24 g carbohydrates | g 2 total fat (.5 g saturated) | 5 mg cholesterol 6 g fiber | 3 g sugar | 280 mg sodium

This recipe is a staple at Mexican carnes asadas (barbecue cookouts) and works equally well with pinto or black beans. To make it into Frijoles Borrachos, blend the garlic, onions, and oregano with 20 ounces of water, instead of 1 quart, and add a 12-ounce bottle of beer to the beans after they have been drained and rinsed. The finished dish should have enough liquid to give it a consistency between that of a stew and a soup, so you may have to add a little more water toward the end; I usually add about ½ cup. For a vegetarian version, omit the bacon and chorizo. In either case, the addition of a little mild vinegar at the end causes the flavor to bloom. I find the salt from the Frijoles de Olla, the bacon, and the chorizo to be enough, but you may want to add a little more at the end with the vinegar. (The nutrition calculations do not include extra salt.)

INGREDIENTS

1 recipe Frijoles de Olla (page 65)
½ tablespoon extra-virgin olive oil
1 slice bacon, finely chopped
1½ ounces (about 3 tablespoons) Mexican chorizo, skinned
    and finely chopped
¾ cup chopped white onion
2 cloves garlic, finely chopped
1 tablespoon finely chopped serrano chile
1 cup crushed canned tomatoes, preferably fire-roasted
½ tablespoon dried leaf oregano
¼ cup loosely packed cilantro
1½ tablespoons rice vinegar

DIRECTIONS

Sauté and add the vegetables. When the Frijoles de Olla are nearly done, heat the olive oil in a skillet over medium heat. Add the bacon and chorizo and cook until most of the fat has rendered. Add the onion, garlic, and chile and continue cooking just until they begin to soften. Add the tomatoes and oregano and continue cooking until the crushed tomatoes begin to thicken and lose their tinny taste, about 5 minutes. Add the cilantro and then pour the contents of the skillet into the beans.

Finish the beans. Add the vinegar and any salt and simmer for 5 minutes.

Frijoles Refritos

REFRIED BEANS

4 half-cup servings

PER SERVING | 200 calories | 8 g protein
24 g carbohydrates | 8 g total fat
(1 g saturated) | 0 mg cholesterol
6 g fiber | 1 g sugar | 240 mg sodium

Refried beans are usually made by frying cooked beans with fat and some of their liquid. The beans are mashed into the liquid with a perforated bean masher as they thicken. The following method, used by many restaurants, avoids that last messy and tedious step by processing the beans with some of their liquid until smooth before adding them to the skillet. The traditional fat is lard, and the only other way to get the right flavor is to use some bacon fat. I sometimes use home-rendered lard, but olive oil also makes a very good substitute. Another delicious option is duck fat. It has fewer calories than olive oil and less saturated fat and cholesterol than other animal fats. The amount of liquid you process the beans with is difficult to specify exactly, but it usually comes to about ½ cup per cup of cooked beans. Just make sure the result is not too thick. If you add a little too much liquid, you just need to cook the beans a little longer to get the right consistency, so err on the side of too much.

INGREDIENTS

2 cups Frijoles de Olla (page 65) made with pinto or black beans, or
    lightly salted or unsalted canned beans, broth reserved
1 cup bean broth
2 teaspoons minced, canned chipotle chile
½ teaspoon ground cumin
½ teaspoon dried leaf oregano
2 tablespoons homemade lard (page 12), extra-virgin olive oil,
    or duck fat
2 cloves garlic, minced
4 teaspoons grated *cotija* cheese (optional; adds fewer than
    10 calories)

DIRECTIONS

Process the beans. Put the beans into a food processor and add the broth, chipotle chile, cumin, and oregano. Process until the beans are smooth, adding more broth if they appear too thick.

Cook the beans. Heat a skillet over medium heat and add the fat or oil. Add the garlic and allow it to cook for just a few seconds, then add the puréed beans. Cook, stirring constantly, until the beans are heated through and as thick or thin as you like them. Serve topped with the cheese, if you wish.

Quick Beans

This recipe produces very good beans in just a few minutes. If you can find them, use canned beans with no added salt.

8 half-cup servings

PER SERVING | 140 calories | 8 g protein
22 g carbohydrates | 3 g total fat
(0 g saturated) | 0 mg cholesterol
8 g fiber | 1 g sugar | 170 mg sodium

INGREDIENTS

3 (14½-ounce) cans black or pinto beans, preferably with no salt added
1 tablespoon extra-virgin olive oil
3 cloves garlic, finely chopped or put through a garlic press
½ heaping teaspoon ground cumin
½ teaspoon dried leaf oregano
½ tablespoon adobo sauce or chopped canned chipotle chile
1 teaspoon rice vinegar
2 tablespoons chopped cilantro
½ teaspoon salt, if using unsalted beans, or to taste

DIRECTIONS

Drain the beans. Drain the liquid from the beans into a bowl and reserve.

Heat the beans. Heat the oil in a medium-sized pot over medium heat, add the garlic, and cook for about 30 seconds; do not allow it to brown. Add the drained beans and the remaining ingredients. Add enough of the reserved bean liquid to achieve whatever consistency you would like and bring the mixture to a simmer. Simmer a minute or 2, and the dish is done.

Santa Maria–style Beans

These unique beans are traditionally served with barbecued meats in Central California. The pinquito variety is found almost nowhere else but around Santa Maria. They are a smaller version of pink beans, which are themselves a smaller version of pinto beans. The latter two are substitutes in that order of preference. Fortunately, pinquitos are available on the Internet and are well worth getting. However, any beans you use will be delicious and a perfect complement to grilled foods. Most California cooks soak the beans, so that is what the recipe calls for.

About 14 half-cup servings

PER SERVING | 160 calories | 9 g protein
23 g carbohydrates | 3.5 g total fat
(1 g saturated) | 5 mg cholesterol
5 g fiber | 2 g sugar | 370 mg sodium

INGREDIENTS

1 pound pinquito beans, or substitute pink or pinto beans
1 tablespoon extra-virgin olive oil
2 pieces of thick-sliced bacon, finely chopped
½ cup lower-sodium ham, cut to a ¼-inch dice
3 cloves garlic, minced
¾ cup crushed tomatoes, preferably fire-roasted
¼ cup Chile Sauce (page 45), or substitute La Palma red chile enchilada sauce; for a more piquant version, use 2 tablespoons sriracha and 2 tablespoons water

1 teaspoon dry mustard

1 tablespoon agave nectar or sugar

1½ teaspoons salt

2 tablespoons minced parsley

Soak the beans. Put the beans in a large strainer or colander, pick them over, and remove any stones or broken beans. Put the beans in a large bowl, cover them by about 2 inches with water, and allow them to soak overnight.

Cook the beans. Drain the beans, place them in a pot, and cover them with water by about 1 inch. Bring to a boil, partially cover the pot, and simmer until they are tender, 45–90 minutes. Check them frequently as you will probably have to add more water from time to time.

Prepare the seasoning sauce. While the beans are cooking, put the olive oil in a skillet over medium heat and add the bacon. When the bacon begins to sizzle, stir in the ham. When the bacon is well browned, add the garlic and cook 1 minute. Stir in the tomatoes, Chile Sauce, mustard, agave nectar, and salt and simmer the sauce until it just begins to thicken, 2–3 minutes.

Finish the beans. When the beans are tender, drain off all but about ½ cup of the liquid and stir in the seasoning sauce. Cook the beans for 1 minute, stir in the parsley, and serve.

RAJAS

Fried or Grilled Strips of Chile and Onion

In culinary terms, *rajas* (pronounced RAH-hahs) refers to sliced chiles and onions that are sautéed or grilled. They are usually served with grilled meats and poultry, such as fajitas, but are also used in tacos and quesadillas, with meat or cheese. For both diet and enjoyment, Rajas make a wonderful accompaniment to grilled beef, pork, lamb, or chicken, often serving as a much more interesting version of "smothered in onions."

There are three basic styles of Rajas. There is the version I call "Seared," where sliced onions and unpeeled poblano chiles are stir-fried in oil over high heat until just cooked through and seared on the outside. Another way of preparing Rajas is to caramelize the onions by cooking them slowly over low heat until they give off nearly all their moisture and become sweet, golden-brown morsels. In that case, the poblanos are always roasted and skinned to produce the proper texture. In some parts of Mexico, including Baja California, the onions and unpeeled chiles are grilled over oak or mesquite, and jalapeños are often used in place of poblanos.

Once the grilled Rajas are cooked, they are sliced or chopped and given a spritz of lime juice. Please note that because they have many fewer onions, the grilled Rajas have fewer carbohydrates.

Seared Rajas

4 servings

PER SERVING | 110 calories | 2 g protein
12 g carbohydrates | 7 g total fat
(1 g saturated) | 0 mg cholesterol
3 g fiber | 6 g sugar | 400 mg sodium

INGREDIENTS

2 tablespoons extra-virgin olive oil
1 medium white onion, cut into ¼-inch slices
2 medium poblano chiles, stemmed, seeded, and cut into ¼-inch slices
¾ teaspoon kosher salt
Freshly ground black pepper, to taste
Juice from ½ lime, or to taste

DIRECTIONS

Heat a 12-inch skillet over medium-high to high heat. Add the olive oil, onions, and chiles, and cook, stirring almost constantly, until the chiles soften, begin to turn golden, and char a bit. Add the salt, pepper, and lime juice, mix well, and serve.

Caramelized Rajas

4 servings

PER SERVING | 150 calories | 3 g protein
21 g carbohydrates | 7 g total fat
(1 g saturated) | 0 mg cholesterol
4 g fiber | 9 g sugar | 410 mg sodium

INGREDIENTS

2 tablespoons extra-virgin olive oil
2 medium white onions, peeled, cut into ¼-inch slices
¾ teaspoon kosher salt
3 cloves garlic, thinly sliced
2 medium poblano chiles, roasted, peeled, seeded, and cut into ¼-inch slices (page 16)
Freshly ground black pepper, to taste
Juice from ½ lime, or to taste

DIRECTIONS

Heat a 12-inch skillet over medium heat. Add the olive oil, onions, and salt, which will help the onions release their liquid. Cook, stirring frequently, until the onions *just* begin to take on color, then reduce the heat to medium-low. Keep cooking the onions slowly, stirring frequently and adjusting the temperature to keep them from scorching, until they are a deep golden brown. Add the garlic and roasted poblano chiles and cook until the garlic and chiles are soft. Stir in the pepper and lime juice and serve.

Grilled Rajas

4 servings

PER SERVING | 30 calories | 1 g protein
7 g carbohydrates | 0 g total fat
(0 g saturated) | 0 mg cholesterol
2 g fiber | 3 g sugar | 260 mg sodium

INGREDIENTS

5 large jalapeño chiles, stemmed, cut in half, and seeded
2 slices (½-inch thick) from the center of a large white onion
3 very large garlic cloves
Cooking spray
½ teaspoon kosher salt
Freshly ground black pepper, to taste
½ teaspoon whole leaf oregano
Juice from ½ lime, or to taste

DIRECTIONS

Prepare the chiles, onion, and garlic. The easiest way to grill the chiles, onions, and garlic is in a perforated steel grill pan. The next best way is to skewer them. To do that, thread the chiles on thin skewers with the cut sides facing the same way. If you use wooden skewers, be sure to soak them to keep them from burning. Pierce the onion slices horizontally with another skewer. Pierce the garlic cloves with another skewer. Spray all the vegetables with cooking spray.

Grill the Rajas. Light a mesquite, oak, or charcoal fire, or turn a gas grill as high as it will go. The best time to grill the Rajas over wood or charcoal is just before the coals are completely ready and there are still some flames. That makes it easy to cook them before you add any meat with which they will be served. Grill the chiles, onions, and garlic until they are golden brown. Some of them will probably become quite charred and blackened, but that's just fine.

Finish the Rajas. Remove the vegetables from the grill, pull them off the skewers, if using, and chop the vegetables coarsely. Toss the Rajas with the salt, pepper, oregano, and lime juice.

Mexican Street Corn

4 servings

PER SERVING | 270 calories | 7 g protein
38 g carbohydrates | 13 g total fat
(2.5 g saturated) | 10 mg cholesterol
5 g fiber | 6 g sugar | 210 mg sodium

One of the joys of walking the streets in Mexico is the sight and aroma of food being prepared in puestos *(stalls), and corn grilling over charcoal or wood coals is one of the best! The following recipe is easy and delicious. The number of calories can be reduced by substituting Miracle Whip for the mayonnaise, if you don't mind the different flavor. You could also use low-calorie mayo. A dusting of* cotija *cheese at the end is optional, but it adds a great deal in return for very few calories.*

INGREDIENTS

**2 tablespoons canola oil
2 cloves garlic, minced or put through a garlic press
4 ears corn, husked
¼ cup mayonnaise
1 teaspoon pure chile powder from ancho or New Mexico chiles
½ teaspoon garlic powder
¼ teaspoon ground cumin
Freshly ground black pepper, to taste
¼ cup grated *cotija* cheese (optional)
Lime wedges**

DIRECTIONS

Prepare the garlic oil. Heat the canola oil over low heat, add the garlic, and sauté until the garlic is soft but not browned.

Grill the corn. Preheat a gas or charcoal grill or a stovetop grill pan. Brush the corn all over with the garlic oil and grill it on all sides over medium to medium-high heat until the corn is tender and well browned, 6–10 minutes.

Prepare the flavoring paste. While the corn is grilling, combine the mayonnaise, chile powder, garlic powder, cumin, and pepper.

Finish the corn. When the corn is done, brush it with the flavoring paste and, if using, dust with the cheese. Serve with the lime wedges.

Roasted-Garlic Sweet Potatoes

4 servings

PER SERVING | 190 calories | 3 g protein
38 g carbohydrates | 3.5 g total fat
(0.5 g saturated) | 0 mg cholesterol
6 g fiber | 7 g sugar | 360 mg sodium

When properly prepared, sweet potatoes can be as good as or better than regular potatoes. They are popular in Mexico, and this recipe, which I adapted from one by Chef Ming Tsai, makes a great side dish. It is also a terrific substitute for both regular roasted potatoes and hash browns and is particularly good with grilled foods and eggs. That the potatoes do not need to be peeled makes the recipe especially easy to prepare. They also heat up well in a microwave, although the crisp texture is lost.

Two important things to remember when making the dish are to cut the potatoes to no more than ½-inch square and to use good oven mitts and extreme caution when extracting the preheated skillet or casserole dish from the oven. I use a 12-inch iron skillet, which decreases the cooking time and makes the potatoes crispier, but you could use any baking dish of the same size.

INGREDIENTS

1½ pounds unpeeled sweet potatoes, cut into ½-inch pieces
12 cloves garlic, peeled and cut in half
1 tablespoon extra-virgin olive oil
1–2 tablespoons minced serrano or jalapeño chile
¾ teaspoon dried thyme
½ teaspoon kosher salt
½ teaspoon pepper

DIRECTIONS

Preheat your oven and pan. Place a 12-inch ovenproof skillet or casserole dish large enough to hold the potatoes in a single layer in the oven, turn the heat to 375°F, and heat the pan for 30 minutes.

Mix the ingredients. While the skillet is heating, combine all the ingredients in a bowl.

Roast the potatoes. Remove the heated skillet from the oven and immediately evenly distribute the mixed ingredients. Put the skillet in the oven and roast the potatoes for 45 minutes, stirring every 15 minutes so they will cook evenly.

Sweet Potatoes Mashed with Coconut Milk and Roasted Garlic

Sweet potatoes are popular in Mexico, especially in tropical areas. This recipe makes a delicious side dish or part of a vegetarian meal, and it does so without resorting to ingredients such as brown sugar and marshmallows. It is also used in the terrific Sweet Potato Enchiladas (page 141).

5 half-cup servings

PER SERVING | 150 calories | 2 g protein
30 g carbohydrates | 2.5 g total fat
(1.5 g saturated) | 0 mg cholesterol
4 g fiber | 6 g sugar | 330 mg sodium

INGREDIENTS

8 cloves garlic, peeled
Cooking spray
½ cup lite coconut milk
1 tablespoon butter substitute, melted
½ tablespoon chopped canned chipotle chile
½ teaspoon salt
1½ pounds sweet potatoes, peeled and cut into 2-inch pieces

DIRECTIONS

Preheat your oven to 350°F.

Roast the garlic and prepare the coconut mixture. Place the garlic on several folds of aluminum foil, spray it liberally with cooking spray, wrap it tightly, and put it in the preheated oven for 45 minutes. Remove the garlic from the oven and, when it is cool enough to handle, unwrap it and put it in the bowl of a food processor. Add the coconut milk, butter substitute, chipotle, and salt and process until thoroughly combined, 30–60 seconds. Reserve.

Cook and finish the sweet potatoes. Put the potatoes in a pot, cover them with water, bring to a boil, and simmer until they are very tender, 10–12 minutes. Drain the potatoes into a strainer and allow them to sit for 3 minutes. Put the potatoes through a potato ricer into a dry bowl, add the coconut mixture, and mix well.

Calabacitas

A savory dish of squash, corn, and mild chiles, Calabacitas is traditionally made with squash, corn, onion, and roasted poblano chiles sautéed in butter, but a good butter substitute works very well. It is best made with fresh corn, but frozen will work in a pinch.

4 servings

PER SERVING | 180 calories | 5 g protein
26 g carbohydrates | 8 g total fat
(2.5 g saturated) | 5 mg cholesterol
4 g fiber | 8 g sugar | 220 mg sodium

INGREDIENTS

3 tablespoons butter substitute
1 cup white onion, sliced about ⅛-inch thick
Kernels from 2 ears of corn, or substitute 1½ cups frozen corn, thawed and measured after thawing
⅔ cup roasted, peeled, and sliced poblano peppers (page 16)

12 ounces zucchini, cut into strips about 2½ inches long
    by ¼-inch wide and thick (about 4 cups)
½ teaspoon dried leaf oregano
¼ teaspoon salt
¼ teaspoon freshly ground black pepper
3 tablespoons sour cream
2 tablespoons loosely packed chopped cilantro

DIRECTIONS

Melt the butter substitute in a pan over medium heat. Add the onion and corn and sauté until the onion is just beginning to soften, about 3 minutes. Add the poblano, zucchini, oregano, salt, and pepper, cover the pan, and cook until the zucchini is soft, about 3 minutes. Add the sour cream and cilantro and toss until well mixed.

Roasted Cauliflower

4 servings

PER SERVING | 110 calories | 4 g protein
10 g carbohydrates | 6 g total fat
(1.5 g saturated) | 0 mg cholesterol
3 g fiber | 3 g sugar | 85 mg sodium

If I could have only one cooked vegetable dish, this might be it. It is easy to prepare, heats up well in a microwave, and is delicious as either a side dish or part of a vegetarian entrée.

INGREDIENTS

1 very large head of cauliflower (about 1 pound 6 ounces after
    trimming), cut into florets 1–3 inches in diameter
1½ tablespoons extra-virgin olive oil
Freshly ground black pepper, to taste
8 cloves garlic, coarsely chopped
2 tablespoons grated *cotija* cheese, or substitute Parmesan

DIRECTIONS

Preheat your oven to 375°F.

Prepare and roast the cauliflower. Arrange the florets in a baking dish that will accommodate them in one layer, stems facing up (I use a 12-inch iron skillet). Add the olive oil, pepper, and half the garlic and toss. Roast for 25 minutes. If the cauliflower has browned on the bottom, turn it so that the browned side is up. If it is not yet brown on the bottom, keep roasting until it is, and then turn it and add the remaining garlic. Lower the heat to 350°F and continue roasting until the cauliflower is tender and well browned, 20–25 minutes, or a total of 45–55 minutes.

Finish the dish. When the cauliflower is tender and golden brown, remove it from the oven and immediately sprinkle on the cheese.

Roasted Carrots

Roasting brings out the best in many vegetables that are otherwise a bit bland, and that is especially true with carrots.

4 servings

PER SERVING | 120 calories | 2 g protein
18 g carbohydrates | 6 g total fat
(1 g saturated) | 0 mg cholesterol
5 g fiber | 8 g sugar | 310 mg sodium

INGREDIENTS

1½ pounds carrots, peeled and cut into ½–¾-inch pieces
6 cloves garlic, peeled and smashed
1½ tablespoons extra-virgin olive oil
¼ heaping teaspoon dried thyme
Freshly ground black pepper, to taste
¼ heaping teaspoon salt

DIRECTIONS

Preheat your oven to 400°F.

Put the carrots in a 12-inch iron skillet or on a baking dish large enough to hold them in a single layer. Stir in the remaining ingredients, cover the skillet tightly with foil, and roast for 30 minutes. Remove the foil and continue roasting for 20 minutes. Stir and roast an additional 5–10 minutes, or until the carrots are well browned.

Pozole Side Dish

Pozole is usually thought of as a stew or soup, where the hominy is just one of several ingredients. However, in New Mexico, pozole is often served as a side dish, sometimes alongside rice and beans, especially on enchilada and combination plates. It is both nutritious and delicious and always reminds me of great meals in Santa Fe, Albuquerque, and Taos. Please see the section on Hominy (page 11) before proceeding.

About 10 servings

PER SERVING | 110 calories | 3 g protein
26 g carbohydrates | 0 g total fat
(0 g saturated) | 0 mg cholesterol
2 g fiber | 1 g sugar | 220 mg sodium

INGREDIENTS

1½ cups dried hominy
½ cup chopped onions
½ cup roasted, peeled, and chopped fresh green New Mexico, Anaheim, or poblano chiles
1 teaspoon dried leaf oregano
¼ cup chopped tomato
¾ teaspoon salt
½ teaspoon freshly ground black pepper

DIRECTIONS

Soak the hominy. The day before you plan to serve the Pozole, put the hominy in a bowl, cover it with several inches of water, and allow it to soak at room temperature for 24 hours.

Cook the Pozole. Drain the hominy and discard the soaking water. Rinse the hominy, put it in a pot, and cover it with 2 inches of water. Bring to a boil, add the remaining ingredients, and simmer, partially covered, until the kernels are al dente and appear about to burst, about 2–2½ hours. Uncover the pot and continue simmering until nearly all the liquid has evaporated.

Savory Corn Fritters

4 servings

PER SERVING | 160 calories | 4 g protein 17 g carbohydrates | 9 g total fat (1.5 g saturated) | 45 mg cholesterol 2 g fiber | 4 g sugar | 230 mg sodium

This is the savory version of sweet Breakfast Corn Cakes (page 224). It leaves the corn kernels whole and adds some chile and spices to make a great accompaniment for poultry or pork. In a pinch, the dish can be made with thawed and towel-dried frozen corn. Each of the chile options creates a different result, and although it is a bit more trouble, I think the roasted poblanos are a bit earthier. Also, please note that if you are using fresh corn, some of the kernels will pop out of the fritters; just use them as a garnish.

INGREDIENTS

¼ cup all-purpose flour

1½ tablespoons cornstarch

½ teaspoon baking powder

¼ teaspoon salt

½ teaspoon dried leaf oregano

¼ teaspoon ground cumin

1 egg, beaten

¼ cup cold water

3 tablespoons roasted, peeled, and finely chopped poblano chile, or substitute 2 tablespoons seeded and finely chopped jalapeño pepper

1½ cups fresh corn kernels (from about 2 ears)

2 tablespoons extra-virgin olive oil

DIRECTIONS

Make the batter. Combine the flour, cornstarch, baking powder, salt, oregano, and cumin. Beat the egg and cold water together and mix thoroughly into the dry ingredients. Stir in the chile and corn and allow the batter to sit for 15–20 minutes to make sure the flour is completely hydrated.

Cook the fritters. Heat a 12-inch nonstick skillet over medium heat (350°–375°F if you have a laser thermometer) and add the oil. Scoop 4 slightly heaping ⅓-cup portions of the batter into the skillet and pat them flat with a spatula. Cook the fritters until they are golden brown on the bottom, about 3 minutes. Turn the fritters and cook until they are browned on the other side, about another 3 minutes.

Calabacitas y Nopalitos

*This cactus-based riff on Calabacitas is one of the best and healthiest side dishes I have ever had, and with the addition of some **queso fresco** it makes an outstanding vegetarian entrée, adding only 60 calories per serving. As a side dish, it goes particularly well with chicken.*

4 servings

PER SERVING | 120 calories | 3 g protein
15 g carbohydrates | 6 g total fat
(1 g saturated) | o mg cholesterol
3 g fiber | 7 g sugar | 160 mg sodium
(calculations do not include the cheese)

INGREDIENTS

1½ tablespoons extra-virgin olive oil

2 cups chopped white onion

1 cup cleaned and chopped nopalitos, ½-inch dice
    (from about ¼ pound)

½ tablespoon butter substitute

1 cup fresh corn kernels (from about 1 ear of corn), or
    substitute thawed frozen corn

1½ cups chopped zucchini, ½–¾-inch pieces

1 teaspoon dried leaf oregano

¼ teaspoon salt

¼ teaspoon freshly ground black pepper

2 tablespoons chopped cilantro

For a vegetarian entrée, 3 ounces *queso fresco*, cut into ¾-inch pieces

DIRECTIONS

Cook the onions and nopalitos. Heat the oil in a large pot or Dutch oven over medium heat, add the onions, and cook, stirring frequently, until they begin to soften, about 2 minutes. Add the nopalitos, cover the pot, and continue cooking for 5 minutes. Uncover the pot. You will see that the nopalitos have released their viscous liquid. To remove it, raise the heat to medium-high and continue cooking, stirring almost constantly, until you see that it has evaporated and the onions are browning. Another signal will be that the crackling and sizzling sound increases; this usually takes 5–7 minutes.

Finish the dish. Add the butter substitute to the pot and melt. Add the corn and cook 1 minute, stirring frequently. Add the zucchini, oregano, salt, and pepper and continue cooking, stirring frequently, until the zucchini is as tender as you like it. Stir in the cilantro and serve, unless you are making the vegetarian entrée. In that case, add the cheese after the cilantro, continue cooking just until the cheese begins to melt, and serve with corn tortillas.

Grilled Prickly Pear Cactus

4 servings

PER SERVING | 25 calories | 1 g protein
4 g carbohydrates | 0.5 g total fat
(0 g saturated) | 0 mg cholesterol
2 g fiber | 1 g sugar | 310 mg sodium

A staple at carnes asadas (cookouts) in northern Mexico, whole grilled prickly pear paddles make an interesting presentation and a delicious accompaniment to grilled meats.

INGREDIENTS

4 medium-sized but thin prickly pear paddles
Salt
Cooking spray

DIRECTIONS

Start a charcoal or wood fire or preheat a gas grill to high.

Prepare the cactus. Remove any spines or nodes from the paddles with a paring knife or the end of a vegetable peeler, using tongs and great care not to be injured by the spines. Cut off and discard about ¼ inch from the perimeter of each paddle. Make parallel slices on the paddles lengthwise about 1 inch apart, from the rounded tops to within about 2 inches of the base of each paddle. Toss the paddles with enough salt to cover both sides and let them sit for 15 minutes in a colander or on a plate.

Grill the cactus. Rinse off the salt, dry the cactus, and liberally spray both sides with cooking spray. Grill on both sides until tender and serve with grilled foods.

Quinoa

About 8 half-cup servings

PER SERVING | 110 calories | 3 g protein
16 g carbohydrates | 4 g total fat
(0.5 g saturated) | 0 mg cholesterol
2 g fiber | 1 g sugar | 160 mg sodium

Quinoa, pronounced KEEN-wah, is originally from South America. Although not usually associated with Mexican cooking, it is included here because it is delicious, is extremely nutritious and easy to prepare, and makes a great substitute for rice and other starches to serve with entrées, especially poultry, fish, and vegetables. Quinoa is very high in protein, and since it contains the essential amino acids, it is a complete protein. It is also fairly high in calcium, making it especially useful for the lactose intolerant. Please note that quinoa comes with a bitter-tasting coating called saponin that is useful for keeping birds and insects from destroying the crop. Be sure to purchase a brand that has removed the coating, or you will have to do that yourself by soaking and rinsing it. ▶▶

For the quinoa

1 cup quinoa

2 cups water

For the dressing

½ teaspoon Dijon mustard

2 teaspoons balsamic vinegar

1 teaspoon agave nectar

¾ teaspoon dried tarragon

⅛ teaspoon freshly ground black pepper

1 tablespoon extra-virgin olive oil

For the vegetables

1 tablespoon butter substitute

¼ cup minced red onion

1 cup diced zucchini, ¼–½-inch pieces

1 tablespoon minced parsley

1 tablespoon minced cilantro

½ teaspoon salt, or to taste

DIRECTIONS

Cook the quinoa. Put the quinoa in a medium-sized saucepan and stir in the water. Bring to a boil, cover, and simmer gently until all the liquid is absorbed, 10–15 minutes.

Make the dressing. While the quinoa is cooking, whisk together the mustard, vinegar, agave nectar, tarragon, and pepper until well combined. Continue whisking as you add the oil in a slow stream.

Sauté the onion and zucchini. Heat a skillet over medium heat. Add the butter substitute and onion and sauté until the onion just begins to soften, about 2 minutes. Stir in the zucchini and continue cooking until it is just tender, 3–4 minutes. Stir in the parsley and cilantro and remove the pan from the heat.

Finish the dish. Combine the quinoa with the onion and zucchini and stir in the dressing. Add salt to taste.

SOUPS

MEXICAN SOUPS range from simple and earthy to elegant and come in an amazing variety.

Sopa Tarasca

TARASCAN SOUP

4 servings

PER SERVING | 290 calories
13 g protein | 26 g carbohydrates
14 g total fat (5 g saturated)
25 mg cholesterol | 5 g fiber
7 g sugar | 490 mg sodium

This traditional soup from the state of Michoacán may be the inspiration for what we now call tortilla soup; if so, it is still one of the very best versions. The cheese increases the amount of sodium but is a delicious addition.

INGREDIENTS

For the tortilla strips
2 corn tortillas, sliced into strips about 2 inches long and ⅛-inch wide
Canola oil for frying the tortilla strips

For the soup
1 tablespoon canola oil
⅔ cup chopped white onions
2 cloves garlic, roughly chopped
2¼ cups canned, unsalted chopped tomatoes with juice
1 tablespoon pure ancho chile powder
Approximately 5 cups low-sodium chicken broth
2 bay leaves
½ teaspoon whole dried thyme
¼ teaspoon marjoram
¼ teaspoon dried leaf oregano
1 teaspoon salt, or to taste
1 cup grated *queso fresco*, or substitute fresh mozzarella
2 ancho chiles, stems and seeds removed, cut in half, and simmered in water for 15 minutes
¼ cup sour cream
1 green onion, minced (green part only)

DIRECTIONS

Fry the tortilla strips. Heat about 2 inches of oil in a medium-sized pot to about 350°F. Fry the tortilla strips until they are crisp. Drain on paper towels and reserve.

Make the soup. Heat a skillet over medium heat, add the oil, and sauté the onions and garlic until the onions are soft but not browned, 4–5 minutes. Place them in a blender, add the tomatoes with their juice and the chile powder, and purée. Add a cup or 2 of broth (whatever your blender will accommodate), pulse to mix, and then pour the mixture into a pot.

Add the remaining broth, the bay leaves, thyme, marjoram, oregano, and salt to the pot. Bring to a boil and simmer for 15 minutes.

Serve the soup. Place ¼ cup of the cheese and ½ soft ancho chile in each of four bowls. Ladle the soup over the cheese and top it with sour cream, tortilla strips, and green onion.

Caldo de Mariscos

SEAFOOD SOUP

~~~~~~~~~~~~~~~~~~~~~~~~~~~~~~

4 servings

PER SERVING | 250 calories | 23 g protein
18 g carbohydrates | 10 g total fat
(1.5 g saturated) | 105 mg cholesterol
4 g fiber | 9 g sugar | 580 mg sodium

This delicious soup, made by reducing tomatoes, onions, carrots, and oregano to a paste, is typical of those served along Mexico's coasts. It can be made with most types of seafood, including fish fillets, scallops, squid, octopus, or crab. However, do try to use some shrimp so that the shells will help make a flavorful broth. Use all fish for a lower sodium count.

INGREDIENTS

½ **pound unpeeled shrimp**
5 **cups low-sodium chicken broth**
1½ **cups clam juice**
3 **cups chopped fresh tomatoes**
4 **cloves garlic, chopped**
1 **serrano chile, stemmed and chopped**
1 **cup chopped white onion**
2 **medium carrots, peeled and chopped**
1 **teaspoon dried leaf oregano**
2 **tablespoons extra-virgin olive oil**
2 **cups diced zucchini or yellow squash (or 1 cup of each),**
    ⅓-inch pieces
¼ **teaspoon salt, or to taste**
¼ **teaspoon freshly ground black pepper, or to taste**
¼ **cup loosely packed chopped cilantro, divided**
½ **pound catfish, or a similar fish**
Lime wedges

DIRECTIONS

Peel the shrimp and flavor the broth. Peel and devein the shrimp under cold running water, reserving the shells. Place the shells in a pot, add the chicken broth, bring to a boil, and simmer for 10 minutes. Remove the pot from the heat, discard the shrimp shells, add the clam juice, and reserve.

Purée the vegetables. Place the tomatoes, garlic, serrano, onion, carrots, and oregano in a blender and purée.

Make the flavoring paste. In a large pot, heat the oil over medium heat and add the vegetable purée. While stirring, gradually raise the heat to medium-high and cook until the paste is reduced to less than a cup and is very thick.

Finish the soup. Remove the pot from the heat and allow the flavoring paste to cool for about 30 seconds. Gradually stir in the broth and bring to a simmer. Add the squash, salt, pepper, and half the cilantro and simmer for 5 minutes. Bring to a full boil over high heat, add the shrimp and catfish, and simmer until just cooked through, usually about when the liquid returns to a boil. Serve the soup immediately with the lime wedges, which are an important addition.

Caldo de Frijoles Negros

4 one-cup soup course servings. For an entrée soup, double the recipe.

PER SERVING | 140 calories | 8 g protein
21 g carbohydrates | 3 g total fat
(0 g saturated) | 0 mg cholesterol
7 g fiber | 2 g sugar | 360 mg sodium

Considering how delicious this soup is, it could not be easier to prepare. If you cannot find an ancho chile, you may substitute 2½ teaspoons pure mild chile powder (preferably made with ancho chiles), but the texture and taste will not be quite as nice. If you can't find low-sodium chicken broth, you will need to make adjustments in the amount of salt you add. If you wish, for extra taste and texture, place ¾ ounce queso fresco in each bowl and ladle the soup over it. This adds about 60 calories per serving but is worth it. If you cannot find unsalted beans, omit the salt or add it to taste.

INGREDIENTS

½ tablespoon extra-virgin olive oil

½ cup chopped white onion

3 cloves garlic, roughly chopped

1 very small ancho chile, seeded and torn into small pieces, or ½ larger chile

1 teaspoon chopped canned chipotle chile

1 (15-ounce) can unsalted black beans, including the liquid

½ teaspoon salt

3 cups low-sodium chicken broth

¼ teaspoon ground cumin

½ tablespoon chopped cilantro

1 sprig epazote (optional)

½ teaspoon smoked sweet Spanish paprika

½ teaspoon salt, if using unsalted beans

¼ teaspoon finely ground black pepper

1 teaspoon freshly squeezed lime juice

1 tablespoon dry sherry

DIRECTIONS

Make the soup. Heat the olive oil in a medium-sized pot over medium heat until it shimmers. Add the onion and cook until it is just soft but not browned. Add the garlic and cook another minute, then add both chiles and continue to cook, stirring frequently, 1½–2 minutes. Add the remaining ingredients except the lime juice and sherry, bring to a boil, partially cover, and simmer for 10 minutes. Allow the mixture to cool. Remove and discard the epazote if you used it. Pour the ingredients into a blender and blend for 2 minutes, or until puréed, in 2 batches if necessary. Return the soup to the pot, bring to a simmer, stir in the lime juice and sherry, and serve.

Caldo Tlapeño

TLAPAN-STYLE SOUP

4 entrée servings,
6–8 as a soup course

PER SERVING | 360 calories
24 g protein | 34 g carbohydrates
14 g total fat (2.5 g saturated)
40 mg cholesterol | 9 g fiber
9 g sugar | 660 mg sodium

This classic Mexican soup is easily made vegetarian by substituting veg-etable broth for chicken broth and medium or hard tofu for the chicken. Although a canned chipotle is listed as an option, this is one place where the dried version works better. If you make the garbanzo beans from scratch and do not add salt, you will reduce the sodium count by about 210 milligrams.

INGREDIENTS

2 tomatoes, broiled (page 17)
6 cups low-sodium chicken broth
½ pound boneless, skinless chicken breasts
1 tablespoon extra-virgin olive oil
1 cup finely chopped white onion
2 cloves garlic, minced
¾ cup peeled and finely chopped carrots
1½ cups canned garbanzo beans, drained and rinsed
1 cup finely chopped zucchini
½ cup frozen green peas, thawed
1 dried chipotle chile, or one canned chipotle plus 1 teaspoon
    adobo sauce
1 teaspoon freshly squeezed lime juice
¼ teaspoon finely ground black pepper
¼ teaspoon salt, or to taste
1 medium ripe avocado, cut into ½-inch pieces
¼ cup grated *cotija* cheese (optional)
Lime wedges

DIRECTIONS

Prepare the tomatoes. Purée the tomatoes in a blender or food processor and strain through the fine blade of a food mill or push them through a strainer. Reserve.

Cook and shred the chicken. Place the broth and chicken breasts in a large pot, bring to a simmer, and cook just until the chicken is cooked through, about 10 minutes. Remove the chicken and reserve the broth. When the chicken has cooled enough to handle, shred it and divide among four soup bowls.

Make the soup. Heat a large pot over medium heat. Add the olive oil and onions and sauté until the onions are just beginning to brown, about 5 minutes. Add the garlic and cook for 1 more minute. Add the reserved broth and the remaining ingredients except the avocado and cheese, and simmer 8–10 minutes.

Finish and serve the soup. Remove the chile and ladle the soup over the cooked chicken. Add equal portions of the avocado to each bowl and top with some of the cheese, if desired. Serve with lime wedges on the side.

Gazpacho

4 servings

PER SERVING | 340 calories | 6 g protein
29 g carbohydrates | 24 g total fat
(3.5 g saturated) | 0 mg cholesterol
6 g fiber | 13 g sugar | 500 mg sodium

Gazpacho is known as a Spanish dish, but it is also very popular in Mexico, where the climate often begs for chilled soup. Too often, gazpacho tastes like a lot of raw vegetables chopped up and served in a bowl of tomato juice, but not this version, which I was told came originally from Andalusia. I particularly like it when both the soup and the croutons are made with whole wheat bread, which adds a hearty, nutty flavor. You can reduce the fat content by using less olive oil, but it will also provide less of the silky texture that makes this gazpacho so special.

INGREDIENTS

2½ pounds tomatoes, cored and chopped
1½ cups cucumber, chopped, peeled, and seeded
1 cup chopped bell pepper, seeds and veins removed
½ jalapeño, stemmed and chopped
⅓ cup chopped red onion
1 large clove garlic, chopped
½ teaspoon salt
½ cup diced whole wheat bread, crusts removed
4 teaspoons sherry vinegar
Pinch ground cumin
⅓ cup plus 1 tablespoon extra-virgin olive oil
1 slice whole wheat bread

DIRECTIONS

"Sweat" the vegetables. Place 2 pounds of the chopped tomatoes, 1 cup of the cucumber, ¾ cup of the bell pepper, the jalapeño, ¼ cup of the red onion, and the garlic in a large bowl and toss with the salt. Finely chop the remaining tomato, cucumber, bell pepper, and onion and reserve for the garnish. Allow the salted vegetables to stand at room temperature for 1 hour.

Soak the bread. At the end of an hour, strain the accumulated juice from the vegetables into a bowl. Add the chopped bread to the juice, let it soak for 1 minute, and put it in a blender.

Make the soup. Add the salted vegetables, vinegar, and cumin to the blender, in two batches if necessary, and purée. If you are puréeing the soup in 1 batch, with the blender running, add ⅓ cup of the olive oil in a thin stream and continue to blend for at least 2 minutes, or until the mixture is completely smooth. If you are making the soup in 2 batches, add half the olive oil to the first batch and the other half to the second. Pour the blended soup into a bowl and stir well. Refrigerate the gazpacho for at least 3 hours or overnight before serving.

Make the croutons. Preheat the oven to 350°F. Brush both sides of the bread with the remaining 1 tablespoon of olive oil, cut it into ½-inch cubes, and bake until firm and toasted, 5–10 minutes.

Serve the gazpacho. Pour the chilled soup into 4 bowls and top with tomato, cucumber, bell pepper, onion, and croutons.

Caldo de Pollo

CHICKEN SOUP

8 half-cup servings

PER SERVING | 210 calories | 27 g protein
11 g carbohydrates | 6 g total fat
(1 g saturated) | 90 mg cholesterol
3 g fiber | 5 g sugar | 540 mg sodium

When Mexicans and Mexican Americans are in the mood for nutritious comfort food, they often turn to chicken soup. Too often, the ingredients are overcooked, making them dry and stringy, especially the chicken and vegetables, or too much fat is left in. This version carefully avoids those problems. There are a fair number of ingredients, but the preparation is quite simple, and the result is a soup filled with a great variety of delicious and good-for-you ingredients. Often some rice or cut ears of corn are included in the soup, but I prefer to put them on the side, with or instead of hot tortillas.

INGREDIENTS

1 cut-up chicken, 4½–5 pounds
1 tablespoon extra-virgin olive or canola oil
1⅓ cups peeled, diced carrots, cut into ½-inch pieces
¾ cup diced celery, ½-inch pieces
1½ cups minced white onion
¼ cup finely chopped, stemmed, and seeded jalapeño pepper
4 cloves garlic, minced
1 tomato, cut into ½-inch pieces
2 tablespoons tomato paste
2 bay leaves
¾ teaspoon dried thyme
¾ teaspoon dried leaf oregano
¾ teaspoon dried marjoram
¼ heaping teaspoon ground cumin
¼ heaping teaspoon dried rubbed sage
¼ teaspoon freshly ground black pepper
2 quarts low-sodium chicken broth
2 cups diced yellow summer squash, ½-inch pieces
2 cups diced zucchini, ½-inch pieces
⅓ cup loosely packed finely chopped cilantro
1 teaspoon salt, or to taste
1½ tablespoons freshly squeezed lime juice
Lime wedges ▸▸

Prep the chicken. Remove the skin from the breast pieces but leave it on the thighs and drumsticks. Heat the oil in a large pot over medium heat, add the thighs and drumsticks skin side down, and fry them until the skins are golden brown, about 8 minutes. Remove the pot from the heat. Place the chicken on a plate and cool. When cool enough to handle, remove and discard the skin.

Begin the soup. Pour off all but 1 tablespoon fat from the pot. Heat the fat over medium heat and add the carrots, celery, onions, and jalapeño. Cook, stirring frequently, until the vegetables are soft, about 10 minutes. Add the garlic and cook for 1 minute. Add the tomato and cook 1 minute. Stir in the tomato paste and cook 1 minute. Stir in the bay leaves, thyme, oregano, marjoram, cumin, sage, pepper, broth, and the thighs and drumsticks. Bring to a boil, cover the pan, and simmer for 10 minutes. Add the breast pieces, cover the pot, and simmer for 25 minutes.

Finish the soup. Remove the pot from the heat and remove all the chicken to a plate. When the chicken is cool enough to handle, remove the meat from the bones and shred or cut it into bite-sized pieces. Bring the soup back to a boil, add both squashes, and simmer, uncovered, for 5 minutes. Add the shredded chicken, cilantro, salt, and lime juice and cook an additional minute.

Serve the soup. Serve with lime wedges and rice, corn on the cob, or hot tortillas.

Caldo Michi

FISH SOUP FROM JALISCO AND MICHOACÁN

4 entrée servings, 8 as a soup course. Nutrition information is for the entrée serving.

PER SERVING | 310 calories | 23 g protein
14 g carbohydrates | 18 g total fat
(3 g saturated) | 70 mg cholesterol
3 g fiber | 8 g sugar | 630 mg sodium

In Mexico this soup is made with both catfish and carp, and usually the whole fish is used to enrich and thicken the broth. Knowing that the traditional recipes have been well chronicled and because my goal is to make these dishes as accessible as possible, I decided to adapt those recipes to make them easier to prepare. Since catfish fillets rather than the whole fish are most often available and because they are much easier to prepare and to eat, I use them and enrich the broth with clam juice. One item that makes the soup distinctive is the use of chiles pickled in homemade vinegar. Several cooks suggest substitutions, and I have found the unripe plums advocated by Patricia Quintana to be my favorite. They work so well that I would not make the recipe without them. Diana Kennedy's recipe calls for vegetable oil, and although it adds 130 calories to each serving, it makes the broth thicker and the dish much richer and more delicious. The tomato can be peeled by putting it in boiling water for 1 minute then into cold water, or with a serrated vegetable peeler, which also works beautifully on the plums.

¼ cup extra-virgin olive oil

1 pound catfish fillets, cut into bite-sized pieces

1 cup chopped white onion

1⅓ cups peeled and chopped tomato

4 cloves garlic, finely chopped

1 teaspoon dried leaf oregano

1½ cups bottled clam juice

4½ cups low-sodium chicken broth

1 cup peeled and chopped carrots

1 cup zucchini, sliced in half lengthwise then cut
    crosswise into ⅛-inch slices

1 cup peeled and finely chopped unripe plums

2 tablespoons minced pickled jalapeños

Scant ½ teaspoon salt, or to taste

1 tablespoon finely chopped fresh basil

2 tablespoons finely chopped cilantro

DIRECTIONS

Sauté the fish. Heat the oil over moderate heat, add the catfish, and cook just until it turns opaque, about 1 minute on each side. Remove the catfish with a slotted spoon to a plate and reserve.

Cook the onions tomato and garlic. Add the onions, tomato, garlic, and oregano to the pot and cook until the onions are soft and the tomatoes well broken down, 5–8 minutes. Add the clam juice, broth, carrots, zucchini, plums, and jalapeños and simmer, covered, for 10 minutes.

Finish the soup. Add the reserved catfish and simmer, uncovered, until the fish is cooked through, about 5 minutes. Stir in the salt, basil, and cilantro and serve.

Sopa de Lima

LIME SOUP

4 servings

PER SERVING | 160 calories
22 g protein | 6 g carbohydrates
4 g total fat (0.5 g saturated)
55 mg cholesterol | 1 g fiber
2 g sugar | 500 mg sodium

Sopa de Lima is the traditional soup of Mexico's Yucatán state, where it is flavored with the area's special limes (Citrus limetta), which are not often found elsewhere in Mexico, much less in the United States. Either Persian or Key lime juices work well as substitutes. Some cooks leave lime slices, including the skin, in the soup, but I think that creates a bitter flavor. Diana Kennedy suggests leaving some lime with skin in the broth for just a few seconds, and you may wish to try that.

The following version is a very simple one, made with packaged chicken broth rather than homemade and with several other shortcuts designed to make the preparation quick and easy. The result is still delicious and perfect for summer dining. In Yucatán, the soup is served garnished with crispy fried tortilla strips. They require a bit more preparation but add a great deal , especially since packaged tortilla chips make a poor substitute. To make them, slice 2 corn tortillas into strips about ¼ inch by 1 ½ inches and fry them in at least an inch of canola oil heated to about 350°F. Using them adds about 50 calories per serving. You can leave the skin on the tomatoes, but the soup is much better without it. All you need to do is put the tomatoes in the simmering broth for 1 minute, cool them under running water, and peel them, or peel them with a serrated vegetable peeler.

INGREDIENTS

¾ pound boneless, skinless chicken breast

6 cups low-sodium chicken broth

2½ teaspoons canola oil

1 tablespoon thinly sliced serrano chile

1 clove minced garlic

½ teaspoon dried oregano

½ cup very finely chopped red onion

1 cup peeled and chopped Roma tomatoes, ¼-inch dice
   (about 2 medium tomatoes)

3 whole allspice berries

½ teaspoon salt

8 teaspoons freshly squeezed lime juice

¼ cup finely chopped cilantro

DIRECTIONS

Cook and shred the chicken. Put the chicken in a pot, cover it with the broth, bring to a boil, and simmer until the chicken is just cooked through, about 10 minutes. Remove the chicken to a plate and allow it cool. Reserve the broth. When the chicken is cool enough to handle, shred it and set aside.

Make the flavoring for the broth. Heat a very small saucepan over medium heat. Add 1 teaspoon of the oil, the serrano chile, garlic, and oregano and cook until the chile and garlic are just soft, 3–4 minutes, but do not allow them to brown. Put the contents of the saucepan into a blender.

Make the broth. When the reserved chicken broth has cooled, add 1 cup to the blender with the broth flavoring and purée. Add as much more of the broth as your blender will comfortably hold and blend briefly to combine.

Make the soup. Heat a pot over medium heat, add the remaining 1½ teaspoons oil, onion, and tomatoes, and sauté until they are just beginning to soften, 3–4 minutes. Add the allspice berries and all of the broth. Stir in the salt and lime juice, bring to a boil, and simmer for 5 minutes.

Serve the soup. Remove the allspice berries and divide the soup among four bowls. Add the tortilla strips, if using them, and the cilantro.

Sopa Poblana

PUEBLA SOUP

4 half-cup servings

PER SERVING | 200 calories
10 g protein | 21 g carbohydrates
9 g total fat (3.5 g saturated)
10 mg cholesterol | 3 g fiber
11 g sugar | 450 mg sodium

This soup manages to be creamy without any cream, and it is a perfect example of rich Puebla-style cooking minus the extra fat and calories. If you want to reduce the calories by another 40 per serving, leave out the cheese. The soup will not be as rich but will still be delicious. If you want more protein, simply add some chopped hard tofu or shredded cooked chicken.

INGREDIENTS

2½ tablespoons butter substitute
4 ounces peeled and chopped potato
3¼ cups low-sodium chicken broth
2 cups thawed frozen corn, measured after thawing
1 cup chopped white onion
2 cups peeled and chopped zucchini
¾ cup roasted, peeled, seeded, and chopped poblano chile (page 16)
¼ heaping teaspoon dried thyme
¼ heaping teaspoon salt
¾ cup 2% milk
2 ounces part skim milk mozzarella

DIRECTIONS

Cook the potatoes and make the broth. Heat a pot over medium heat. Melt ½ tablespoon of the butter substitute and add the potatoes. Sauté the potatoes until they are beginning to soften, but do not allow them to brown, 4–5 minutes. Add 1¼ cups broth to the pot, cover, and simmer for 5 minutes. Pour the broth and potatoes into a blender, add ½ cup of the corn, and blend until the corn is puréed, about 2 minutes. Add the remaining broth and pulse to combine.

Cook the vegetables. Over medium heat, melt the remaining butter substitute in the same pot in which you cooked the potatoes. Stir in the onions and zucchini and cook until the onions are soft but not browned, about 5 minutes. ▸▸

Make the soup. Add the rest of the corn, the chiles, thyme, salt, and blended potatoes and broth to the vegetables and simmer for 5 minutes. Stir in the milk and simmer for another 5 minutes. Add the cheese and immediately remove the pot from the heat. Stir until the cheese has melted, about 1 minute.

SALADS

UNFORTUNATELY, most Mexican restaurants in the United States don't go much beyond a Caesar or taco salad, but south of the border there are many more delicious options.

Ensalada de Papas

POTATO SALAD

4 servings. Nutrition information includes the avocado.

PER SERVING | 260 calories | 6 g protein
26 g carbohydrates | 15 g total fat
(2.5 g saturated) | 10 mg cholesterol
6 g fiber | 4 g sugar | 300 mg sodium

Served warm or at room temperature, this potato salad goes beautifully with fried dishes, tortas (sandwiches), and anything else with which you would normally serve potato salad. The small amount of chorizo goes a long way in terms of flavor. The recipe can be made with or without the avocado to create two very different experiences, both of which are excellent. The salad can be made well in advance and warmed in a microwave, but do not add the avocado until you are ready to serve.

INGREDIENTS

For the dressing
½ tablespoon rice vinegar
½ teaspoon Dijon mustard
⅛ teaspoon salt
¼ teaspoon pepper
2 tablespoons extra-virgin olive oil
1 tablespoon finely chopped chives
1 tablespoon finely chopped parsley
1 tablespoon finely chopped cilantro

For the salad
1¼ cups peeled diced carrots, ½-inch pieces
2½ cups peeled and diced potatoes, ½-inch pieces
2 ounces chorizo, skin removed, finely chopped
1 serrano chile, seeds and veins removed, minced
1 medium to large avocado, cut into ½-inch pieces (optional)

DIRECTIONS

Make the dressing. In a bowl, whisk together the vinegar, mustard, salt, and pepper. Add the olive oil in a slow stream, whisking constantly to create an emulsion, then add the chives, parsley, and cilantro and mix well.

Cook the potatoes and carrots. Bring 6 cups of water to a boil. Add the salt and carrots and simmer until the carrots are very tender but not mushy. Remove the cooked carrots with a strainer and rinse under cold running water to stop the cooking. Cook the potatoes in the same water until very tender but not mushy and drain in a colander. Rinse under cold running water to stop the cooking.

Cook the chorizo. Heat a nonstick skillet over medium heat and add the chorizo. As soon as it starts to sizzle, add the serrano and continue cooking, stirring and breaking up the chorizo with a plastic or wooden spoon, until it is golden and beginning to crisp.

Finish the salad. When the chorizo is done, remove the skillet from the heat. Let it cool for 1 minute then stir in the reserved carrots and potatoes. Scrape everything into a medium-sized bowl, add the dressing and the avocado, if using, and mix gently but thoroughly.

Naturally Healthy Mexican Cooking

Ensalada Tequilero

TEQUILA-MAKER'S SALAD

4 servings

PER SERVING | 460 calories
15 g protein | 39 g carbohydrates
29 g total fat (7 g saturated)
20 mg cholesterol | 10 g fiber
10 g sugar | 550 mg sodium

The word tequilero *refers to a person who makes or sells tequila. The recipe gets its name from the fact that part of the dressing is made with* sangrita, *which is usually drunk as a chaser with tequila, probably the most popular way to drink it in Mexico. The salad is easy to prepare and makes a terrific lunch or supper. Please see the Ingredients section for instructions for preparing the nopalitos (page 12). If you make the garbanzo beans from scratch and do not add any salt, you will lower the sodium for each serving by over 200 milligrams.*

INGREDIENTS

For the dressing

2 tablespoons *sangrita* (page 28)

1 tablespoon plus 2 teaspoons freshly squeezed lime juice

1 teaspoon Dijon mustard

¼ cup extra-virgin olive oil

Salt to taste (I add none because of the salt in the beans and nopalitos if I'm using canned ones)

¾ teaspoon freshly ground black pepper, or to taste

For the salad

2 cups cooked fresh corn, frozen corn in a pinch

1 cup nopalitos, preferably homemade cured in salt or boiled until tender (canned may be used if you adjust for their high salt content [pages 12–14])

2 cups canned garbanzo beans, rinsed and drained

2 cups fresh spinach, packed

1 large tomato, cut into bite-sized pieces

1 large avocado or 2 small ones, chopped

2 green onions, finely chopped

¼ cup minced cilantro

4 ounces *queso fresco*

DIRECTIONS

Make the dressing. In a small to medium-sized bowl, whisk together the *sangrita*, lime juice, and mustard. Continue whisking vigorously as you add the olive oil in a slow stream, until the dressing emulsifies. Stir in the salt and pepper.

Make the salad. Combine all of the salad ingredients in a large bowl. Add the dressing and toss well.

Ensalada Caesar

CAESAR SALAD

4 entrée servings

PER SERVING | 330 calories | 7 g protein
15 g carbohydrates | 28 g total fat
(5 g saturated) | 50 mg cholesterol
4 g fiber | 2 g sugar | 400 mg sodium

Growing up in California, about thirty miles north of Tijuana, I was able to sample the original Caesar salad at the original restaurant on Avenida Revolución many times. Over the years, I have tried different versions and have finally settled on the following recipe, which I think is even better than the original. Specific differences are the use of a coddled rather than a raw egg for what to me is a more pleasant taste and consistency, the use of anchovy paste rather than whole anchovies for convenience, the addition of hot sauce, a little Dijon mustard for flavor and to help emulsify the dressing, and the addition of avocado, which pairs perfectly with the other ingredients. At Caesar's, they had room-temperature bottles of olive oil and garlic to make the salads. I did that too until I learned that leaving a mixture of olive oil and garlic for any length of time, especially at room temperature, can cause the growth of deadly botulism bacteria. I now leave a few cloves of smashed fresh garlic in extra-virgin olive oil at room temperature for just 3 hours before making the salad, and it works just as well. I particularly like nuovo, or unfiltered, olive oil because of its robust flavor.

INGREDIENTS

For the garlic-infused olive oil
5 tablespoons robust extra-virgin olive oil
3 cloves garlic, peeled and smashed

For the dressing
1 large egg
¼ teaspoon anchovy paste, or to taste
¼ teaspoon salt
Freshly ground black pepper, to taste
½ teaspoon Dijon mustard
½ teaspoon Worcestershire sauce
¼ teaspoon sriracha or Tabasco sauce
1 tablespoon freshly squeezed lime juice

For the croutons
1 slice bread
1 tablespoon garlic-infused oil

For the salad
7–8 ounces romaine lettuce, sliced crosswise into 1-inch ribbons
1 large avocado, diced
⅓ cup grated Parmesan cheese

Preheat your oven to 350°F.

Infuse the olive oil. No more than 3 hours before preparing the salad, combine the olive oil and garlic and leave at room temperature.

Make the dressing. To coddle the egg, immerse it in boiling water for 30 seconds, remove it immediately and break it into the salad bowl before it overcooks. Add the anchovy paste, salt, pepper, mustard, Worcestershire sauce, sriracha, and lime juice and whisk until thoroughly combined. Remove the garlic from the oil and reserve 1 tablespoon oil for the croutons. Slowly whisk the remaining 4 tablespoons oil into the other dressing ingredients.

Make the croutons. Brush both sides of the bread with the reserved tablespoon of the flavored oil, cut it into 1-inch pieces, and bake until they turn golden brown.

Make the salad. Toss the lettuce and avocado with the dressing and 2 tablespoons of the cheese. Divide the salad among four serving plates, top with shrimp or chicken, if using, and garnish with the remaining cheese.

Ensalada de Col

COLESLAW

PER SERVING | 70 calories | 1 g protein
6 g carbohydrates | 5 g total fat
(0 g saturated) | 0 mg cholesterol
2 g fiber | 2 g sugar | 350 mg sodium

Coleslaw is usually made with either a creamy or vinaigrette dressing. Because it goes so well with Mexican food, my favorite is the vinaigrette version served with combination plates at Tony's Jacal, just north of Del Mar, California. The following is an adaptation of their recipe. You can use all green or all purple cabbage, but for the visual contrast I prefer the proportions in the recipe. Do not be concerned with the amount of salt. It is used to "cure" the slaw and then much of it is poured off with the excess dressing. It is difficult to measure the remaining salt, so if sodium is a serious consideration for you, please use your own judgment.

INGREDIENTS

For the dressing
2 tablespoons plus 2 teaspoons cider vinegar
2 teaspoons salt
½ teaspoon finely ground black pepper
⅓ cup canola oil

For the slaw
12 ounces very finely sliced or shredded green cabbage
6 ounces very finely sliced or shredded purple cabbage
4 ounces peeled shredded carrots ▸▸

Make the dressing. Whisk together the vinegar, salt, and pepper, and then whisk in the oil in a slow stream.

Make the slaw. Combine the slaw ingredients in a large bowl and toss with the dressing. Leave the slaw at room temperature for 3 to 4 hours, stirring it about every half hour. At the end of that time, the cabbage will have softened and the flavors melded. Pour the slaw into a large strainer to drain the excess liquid (and salt) and refrigerate until ready to serve, pouring off any excess liquid from time to time. The slaw keeps, refrigerated, for about a week.

Ensalada de Camarones

SHRIMP SALAD

4 entrée servings, or 6 as an appetizer

PER SERVING | 290 calories
18 g protein | 17 g carbohydrates
18 g total fat (2.5 g saturated)
145 mg cholesterol | 6 g fiber
6 g sugar | 420 mg sodium

I first sampled this salad many years ago in Acapulco and later as a shrimp cocktail in Peru. Tender chilled shrimp are mixed with chopped tomato and avocado in a tangy Thousand Island dressing that is a welcome change from the usual red cocktail sauce. I make it with a combination of regular mayonnaise and Miracle Whip. If you like it well enough and want even fewer calories, use all Miracle Whip, which has only 40 percent as many calories as mayo. Please note that it takes about 1 ½ pounds unpeeled frozen shrimp to make 1 pound after thawing and peeling.

INGREDIENTS

For the dressing
2 tablespoons mayonnaise
2 tablespoons Miracle Whip
2 tablespoons catsup
1 tablespoon sweet pickle relish
1 teaspoon salsa (such as Valentina, Tabasco, or sriracha)
½ teaspoon Worcestershire sauce
½ teaspoon coarsely ground black pepper

For the salad
1 pound large (21–25 per pound) fresh shrimp, peeled
1 cup chopped tomato
2 cups chopped avocado (about 2 large)
1 green onion, minced

Make the dressing. Stir together the mayonnaise, Miracle Whip, catsup, relish, salsa, Worcestershire sauce, and pepper in a small bowl.

Prepare the shrimp. Bring a large pot of water to a boil, add the shrimp, and return to a boil. The shrimp should just be turning pink. Immediately immerse them in ice water to keep them from overcooking.

Make the salads or cocktails. Combine the chilled and towel-dried shrimp with the tomato, avocado, and green onion. Add the dressing and toss well.

Ensalada de Salmón Ahumado

SMOKED SALMON SALAD

4 servings

PER SERVING | 480 calories
37 g protein | 11 g carbohydrates
34 g total fat (7 g saturated)
95 mg cholesterol | 7 g fiber
2 g sugar | 910 mg sodium

This recipe uses the same combination of ingredients as the Smoked Salmon Tacos (page 128), with an entirely different but just as delicious result.

INGREDIENTS

For the spinach bed
½ tablespoon sherry vinegar
⅛ teaspoon salt
⅛ teaspoon freshly ground black pepper
2 tablespoons extra-virgin olive oil
3 ounces fresh spinach leaves

For the salad
1 recipe Smoked Salmon with Truffled Avocado Sauce (page 114)
3 ounces goat cheese
1 recipe Mango Salsa (page 40)

DIRECTIONS

Make the spinach bed. Whisk the vinegar in a medium-sized bowl with the salt and pepper. Still whisking, gradually add the olive oil. Add the spinach and toss well with the dressing. Make a bed of dressed spinach on each of four plates.

Make the salad. Mound equal portions of the Smoked Salmon with Truffled Avocado Sauce over the spinach and top with equal portions of goat cheese and Mango Salsa.

Salpicón de Jaiba

CRAB SALPICÓN

4 servings

PER SERVING | 330 calories
22 g protein | 12 g carbohydrates
22 g total fat (3.5 g saturated)
90 mg cholesterol | 5 g fiber
5 g sugar | 680 mg sodium

The dictionary defines the word salpicón *as "chopped seafood or meat with onion, tomato, and peppers." That comes nowhere near describing how good this dish is. I have had seafood* salpicón *in Veracruz and beef* salpicón *in Chihuahua. Although each one is distinctive, it is difficult to say which is better. Both of them deliver a reward that you can look forward to without sweating the calories. For this one, just be sure you get the finest lump crabmeat available.*

INGREDIENTS

For the dressing

2 tablespoons freshly squeezed lime juice
2 tablespoons sherry vinegar
¼ teaspoon salt
½ teaspoon freshly ground black pepper
¼ cup extra-virgin olive oil

For the salpicón

1 pound top-quality lump crabmeat
¼ cup sliced manzanilla olives
2 green onions, finely chopped
¼ cup sliced red onion, ⅛-inch thick and ½-inch long
½ cup roasted, peeled, and chopped poblano chile (page 16)
1 large avocado, chopped
½ cup diced Roma tomato, ¼–½-inch dice
¼ cup finely chopped cilantro
2 cups fresh spinach

DIRECTIONS

Make the dressing. In a small bowl, whisk together the lime juice, vinegar, salt, and pepper. Continue whisking vigorously as you add the olive oil in a slow stream.

Make the salpicón. Put the crab, olives, green and red onions, poblano, avocado, tomato, cilantro, and spinach in a large salad bowl, pour in the dressing, and toss very gently with a large spoon, breaking up the crabmeat as little as possible. Refrigerate the *salpicón* for an hour, gently turning it every 20 minutes.

Salpicón de Carne de Res

BEEF SALPICÓN

4 servings

PER SERVING | 340 calories
16 g protein | 14 g carbohydrates
26 g total fat (7 g saturated)
30 mg cholesterol | 5 g fiber
6 g sugar | 510 mg sodium

This is my favorite beef salpicón, and it is similar to one of the most popular offerings at Julio's Café Corona in El Paso, Texas (formerly located in Ciudad Juárez), except for the olives. It has a hearty beef flavor without much fat, and the spicy, tart dressing blends beautifully with the richness of the meat and avocados. Once you've made the Carne Seca, it's a snap.

INGREDIENTS

For the dressing

2 tablespoons rice vinegar

⅛ teaspoon salt

¼ teaspoon freshly ground black pepper

¼ teaspoon dried leaf oregano

1 clove garlic, minced

2 tablespoons extra-virgin olive oil

For the salad

3 cups Carne Seca filling (page 116)

1 tablespoon rinsed, seeded, minced canned chipotle pepper

2 green onions, finely sliced crosswise

⅓ cup sliced black California olives

1 cup chopped tomato

1 large avocado, chopped

2 ounces part skim milk mozzarella, grated

⅓ cup roasted, peeled, and sliced poblano chiles (page 16)

½ cup loosely packed chopped cilantro

4 cups sliced lettuce

4 teaspoons grated *cotija* cheese

DIRECTIONS

Make the dressing. Whisk together the vinegar, salt, pepper, oregano, and garlic in a small bowl. Continue whisking as you add the olive oil in a slow stream.

Make the salad. Gently combine the remaining ingredients except the lettuce and *cotija* cheese. Add the dressing and mix. Make a bed of lettuce on each of four plates. Mound equal portions of the mixed ingredients onto the lettuce, sprinkle on the cheese, and serve.

Ensalada de Frutas

FRUIT SALAD

4 servings

PER SERVING | 150 calories | 3 g protein
38 g carbohydrates | 0 g total fat
(0 g saturated) | 0 mg cholesterol
7 g fiber | 31 g sugar | 0 mg sodium

This is my favorite fruit salad, and it could not be easier. I had the original in the state of Michoacán, which is known for its fruterías *and* licuado *(smoothie) stands. I love the tart dressing, but it is easily sweetened with the addition of a little more agave nectar, which costs very few calories (20 per teaspoon). The recipe is purposely simple, designed to provide the basis for your own inspiration. Choose whichever of your favorite fruits are freshest and, if you like, add a little chopped fresh mint or the green part of green onions. When in a hurry, I am particularly fond of the combination of bananas and canned pineapple. When time permits, I love to take advantage of the large number of formerly difficult-to-find tropical fruits that are now much more readily available. The recipe is for a medium-sized salad. Doubling the ingredients and adding a little* queso fresco, *feta, or even cottage cheese makes a satisfying entrée. You also might add a few chopped nuts and some chile powder to the dressing.*

INGREDIENTS

4½ tablespoons freshly squeezed lime juice
1½ tablespoons agave nectar or honey
6 cups chopped fresh fruit

DIRECTIONS

Combine the lime juice and agave nectar or honey and toss with the fruit and any additional ingredients you fancy.

EGG DISHES

As with nearly everything else, Mexicans have developed new and delicious ways of preparing eggs.

Huevos Motuleños

MOTUL-STYLE EGGS

4 servings

PER SERVING | 450 calories
24 g protein | 42 g carbohydrates
21 g total fat (4.5 g saturated)
385 mg cholesterol | 8 g fiber
9 g sugar | 640 mg sodium

My favorite Mexican egg dish is Huevos Motuleños, from the town of Motul, just northeast of Mérida in Yucatán state. Whenever I have them I'm transported to casual cafés where the tropical breeze is only partially cooled by ceiling fans. The dish takes a little effort and timing, but most of the ingredients can be prepared in advance. The refried beans used in Huevos Motuleños are often made with frijoles colados, *black beans that have been strained before being fried, but making refried beans from our Quick Beans (page 68) recipe works well.*

Traditionally, the corn tortillas are fried in a little oil at about 350°F, just long enough so that they just begin to harden. While I use the microwave to soften corn tortillas for enchiladas, when you give them enough time to become a bit stiffer, they become tough. Putting the sprayed tortillas on oven racks in a 350° oven for about 4 minutes works fairly well, but do not leave them much longer or they will also be tough and difficult to cut. The nutrition information is based on the oven method. The neatest way to fry the eggs is with egg molds, thin steel circles about the size of a corn tortilla that keep two eggs together and perfectly round.

INGREDIENTS

8 corn tortillas

Cooking spray for softening the tortillas and frying the eggs

1 cup Refried Black Beans (page 67) or made from the Quick Beans recipe

8 eggs, with 2 each broken into 4 small cups

1 cup Yucatán-style Tomato Salsa (page 49)

1 cup frozen green peas, simmered in water for about 1½ minutes, drained and reserved

3 ounces of low-sodium ham, cut into ¼-inch dice

2 tablespoons grated *cotija* cheese

DIRECTIONS

Prepare the tortillas. Cook the tortillas until they are just beginning to harden but not crisp. Do this either by passing them through hot oil or by baking them as described above. Place 1 cooked tortilla on each of four serving plates, reserving the other 4 tortillas. If not already hot, heat the beans in a microwave and spread ¼ cup of them on top of each tortilla on the plates.

Cook the eggs and finish the dish. Spray 1 or 2 nonstick skillets with cooking spray and heat over medium heat. Fry the eggs 2 at a time until they are done as you like them. Traditionally, they are served sunny-side up. Place 2 cooked eggs on the beans and cover with the remaining tortillas. Spoon some of the salsa on each egg "sandwich," and top with equal amounts of the peas, ham, and cheese.

Naturally Healthy Mexican Cooking

Tortilla Española

SPANISH-STYLE OMELET

4 servings

PER SERVING | 290 calories | 10 g protein
18 g carbohydrates | 20 g total fat
(4 g saturated) | 235 mg cholesterol
2 g fiber | 3 g sugar | 170 mg sodium

This version of the famous Spanish tortilla—actually a very special kind of omelet—is loosely based on one I found in The New Spanish Table *by Anya Von Bremzen. It is especially good served with aioli or, as it is called in Spain, allioli. It heats up well and is also very good at room temperature. Turning the omelet takes a little bit of dexterity but is well worth the effort. Jars of roasted and peeled* piquillo *peppers are available in most supermarkets.*

INGREDIENTS

4 tablespoons extra-virgin olive oil
1¼ cups chopped onions
10 ounces russet potatoes, peeled and cut into ½ inch pieces
5 large eggs (about 9 ounces after shelling)
⅛ heaping teaspoon salt
Freshly ground black pepper, to taste
⅓ cup roasted and peeled *piquillo*, red bell, or poblano peppers, chopped

DIRECTIONS

Cook the vegetables. Heat 2 tablespoons of the oil in a nonstick skillet over medium heat until it shimmers. Add the onions and cook until they are soft, turning down the heat if necessary to keep them from browning. Add the potatoes, lower the heat to medium-low, and cook, turning frequently, until the potatoes are soft but not browned. Remove the potato-onion mixture to a bowl and allow it to cool.

When the potato mixture has cooled, add the eggs, salt, pepper, and the roasted pepper.

Cook the omelet on the first side. Heat a 9-inch skillet over medium-high heat. Add the remaining 2 tablespoons oil, and as soon as it begins to smoke, add the egg mixture. Turn the heat down to medium-low and allow the mixture to cook until it is nearly but not completely set, occasionally shaking the pan. There will still be some liquid on the top, but not enough to quickly run out when the omelet is turned.

Cook the omelet on the second side. Remove the skillet from the heat and run a thin spatula around the edges of and underneath the omelet to make sure it will not stick to the pan. Place a plate slightly larger than the skillet on top of the skillet and, using oven mitts, quickly flip the skillet so that the omelet lands on the plate. Slide the omelet back into the skillet, cooked side up, and continue cooking for about 4½ minutes, or until the eggs are firm and cooked through. Flip the omelet onto a plate and allow it to set for 5 minutes before serving.

Huevos Tirados

TOSSED EGGS

~~~~~~

4 servings

PER SERVING | 310 calories | 18 g protein
24 g carbohydrates | 15 g total fat
(4.5 g saturated) | 280 mg cholesterol
8 g fiber | 2 g sugar | 460 mg sodium

The name Huevos Tirados probably comes from the fact that the eggs are only partially cooked before the black beans are added, and then the ingredients are tossed, or thrown, together. In any case, they make a terrific breakfast or brunch and can literally be thrown together in just a few minutes. The amount of salt depends on how much sodium the beans have. I usually use canned beans with no salt added, and that is what the recipe calls for. The same goes for the amount of liquid added to the beans. They should be runnier than finished refried beans but not so runny that they do not hold together. Because it is important not to overcook the eggs, the recipe calls for heating the beans before they are added to the eggs. For me the easiest way to do that is to use a microwave, but they could also be heated on the stove.

INGREDIENTS

For the beans

1 tablespoon extra-virgin olive oil

⅔ cup finely chopped white onion

4 teaspoons finely chopped jalapeño chile

1 clove garlic, finely chopped

2 cups cooked black beans, cooking liquid reserved

¾ cup liquid from the beans

½ teaspoon ground cumin

½ teaspoon dried leaf oregano

¼ teaspoon salt, or to taste

For the eggs

¼ teaspoon salt, or to taste

¼ teaspoon ground black pepper

6 large eggs

2 tablespoons butter substitute

1½ tablespoons grated *cotija* cheese

DIRECTIONS

Prepare the beans. Heat a skillet over medium heat, add the olive oil, onions, and jalapeño, and cook, stirring frequently, until the onion is soft and just beginning to brown. Add the garlic and cook 1 minute. Put the onion mixture into the bowl of a food processor, add the beans, about ½ cup of their liquid, the cumin, oregano, and salt, and purée. If necessary, add enough more bean liquid so that the beans are a little runnier than you want them to be when finished. Place the beans in a microwave-safe bowl and reserve.

Finish the dish. Stir the salt and pepper into the eggs and beat them until the yolks and whites are well combined. Just before you cook the eggs, heat the beans in the microwave until they are very hot. Heat a skillet over medium heat, add the butter substitute, and when it has melted, pour in the eggs. Using a large spoon or heatproof rubber spatula, stir the eggs using large, sweeping strokes. Just as the eggs come together and begin to solidify, fold the beans into them. Because the eggs will continue to cook after you remove them from the pan, serve the Huevos Tirados as soon as they appear to be cooked through and firm. Sprinkle some of the cheese over each portion and serve.

Ojos de Buey

EYES OF THE OX

4 servings

PER SERVING | 320 calories | 17 g protein
23 g carbohydrates | 17 g total fat
(4.5 g saturated) | 375 mg cholesterol
3 g fiber | 2 g sugar | 810 mg sodium

The name of this delicious Old Spanish California dish comes from the fact that the egg yolks resemble the eyes of an ox, which makes a great presentation. For 2 servings I use an iron skillet about 7 inches in diameter, measured at the bottom, and for 4 servings, a 9-inch one. For a great presentation you could also use individual baking dishes about 5 inches in diameter.

INGREDIENTS

8 large eggs
2 cups Chile Sauce (page 45)
Cooking spray
4 corn tortillas
1 cup pitted and sliced black California olives
2 tablespoons grated *cotija* cheese
2 tablespoons minced parsley

DIRECTIONS

Preheat your oven to 350°F.

Ready the eggs. Break 2 eggs each into 4 small dishes.

Cook the eggs. Bring the Chile Sauce to a boil, remove it from the heat, and allow it to cool for 1 minute. Spray the bottom of the skillet or baking dishes with cooking spray and pour in the Sauce. Carefully put each serving of 2 eggs into the skillet or baking dishes with the Chile Sauce, place them in the oven, and bake until the eggs are set, 8–12 minutes.

Serve the eggs. While the eggs are cooking, spray the tortillas on both sides with cooking spray, wrap them in a towel or place them in a tortilla warmer, and microwave for about 40 seconds.

Just before serving, place a softened tortilla on each of four small plates. With a spatula, carefully place a pair of eggs on the tortilla and spoon the rest of the Chile Sauce around the edges. If using individual baking dishes, serve the tortillas on the side. In either case, place a piece of sliced olive in the center of each yolk to resemble the ox's eyeball and the rest of them around the edge of the sauce. Sprinkle on the cheese and garnish with the parsley.

Chilaquiles Sencillos

4 servings

PER SERVING | 280 calories
16 g protein | 12 g carbohydrates
18 g total fat (6 g saturated)
375 mg cholesterol | 0 g fiber
1 g sugar | 480 mg sodium

Chilaquiles usually consist of things like eggs, meat or poultry, and, often, leftovers, all tossed with crispy little bits of tortilla chips and salsa and topped with cheese. Not only do they invite creativity but they are also one of the most underutilized dishes in Mexican restaurants. They are usually served for breakfast or brunch and sometimes as a side dish. Although the following recipe is probably the easiest you'll find anywhere, it will get raves from friends and family in return for just a few minutes of preparation. Use any mild salsa, red or green. My favorites are the Ancho and Chile de Árbol Salsa (page 43), the Chile Sauce (page 45), or the Fresh Tomatillo Salsa (page 39), which imparts a delicious citrusy flavor. You can make the chips from scratch or use packaged ones, preferably unsalted. While this recipe is designed to show how easy the dish can be, you can certainly make it even better by sautéing some onion and maybe some chopped ham or chorizo before adding the eggs and adding some minced cilantro or chives to the eggs.

INGREDIENTS

2 tablespoons butter substitute
8 large eggs, beaten until smooth
¼ teaspoon salt
1⅓ cups (about 1½ ounces) fried tortilla chips, either fried at home from tortillas cut into strips ¼-inch wide by 1½-inches long or purchased chips crushed into small pieces
1–1¼ cups mild salsa, red or green
¼ cup grated *cotija* cheese

DIRECTIONS

Place the butter substitute in a large nonstick skillet over medium heat. When it is melted, add the eggs and salt and begin stirring and folding them in long, sweeping motions. As soon as the eggs begin to solidify, add the tortilla chips and salsa and continue stirring until the eggs are done as you like them. Sprinkle 1 tablespoon of cheese over each serving.

Huevos Rancheros

~~~~~~~~~~~~~~~~~~~~~~~~~~~~~~~~

4 servings

PER SERVING | 350 calories | 15 g protein
30 g carbohydrates | 15 g total fat
(5 g saturated) | 375 mg cholesterol
9 g fiber | 0 g sugar | 640 mg sodium

Huevos Rancheros is probably the most popular Mexican egg dish and comes in countless variations. It consists of semicrisp corn tortillas topped with fried eggs that are usually covered with a tomato-based Ranchero Sauce. Sometimes a green chile sauce is used, especially in New Mexico. As with the Huevos Motuleños recipe, to reduce calories and fat, I suggest that the tortillas be prepared by spraying them on both sides with cooking spray then baking them for a few minutes. The dish is usually served with Refried Beans alongside the eggs and tortillas or under the eggs on the tortillas.

INGREDIENTS

4 corn tortillas
Cooking spray
8 large eggs
2 cups Refried Beans (page 67), heated
2 cups Ranchero Sauce (page 39), heated
¼ cup *cotija* cheese
3 tablespoons chopped cilantro

DIRECTIONS

Preheat your oven to 350°F.

Cook the tortillas. Spray the tortillas on both sides with cooking spray, put them on a rack in the oven, and bake until they just begin to harden, about 4 minutes. Remove the tortillas and place them on serving plates.

Cook the eggs. Break 2 eggs each into 4 small bowls. Heat a large nonstick skillet over medium heat, spray it with cooking spray, and put in each pair of eggs, using circular egg molds, if you wish. You will probably have to do this in two batches.

Finish the dish. Place equal portions of the beans either on the tortillas or on one side of them. When the eggs are done as you like them, place each pair on top of a tortilla (or the tortilla and beans). Top each pair of eggs with a half cup of Ranchero Sauce, and then garnish with the cheese and cilantro.

Huevos Beneficiosos

BENEFICIAL EGGS

4 servings

PER SERVING | 410 calories | 23 g protein
30 g carbohydrates | 22 g total fat
(9 g saturated) | 215 mg cholesterol
4 g fiber | 6 g sugar | 600 mg sodium

Using the delicious and nutritious Romesco Sauce instead of hollandaise, this dish produces a healthy Mexican answer to Eggs Benedict. The eggs can also be placed on halved English muffins instead of the tortilla sandwiches, if you wish.

INGREDIENTS

4 ounces part skim milk mozzarella cheese

8 corn tortillas

2 poblano chiles, roasted, peeled, and cut in half (page 16)

4 ounces thinly sliced low-sodium ham

Cooking spray

4 large eggs

½ cup Romesco Sauce (page 50)

DIRECTIONS

Form the tortilla "sandwiches." Sprinkle ½ ounce cheese on each of 4 tortillas, top them with equal portions of the chiles and ham, and add the remaining ½ ounce cheese. Top with the last 4 tortillas and reserve.

Cook the tortilla "sandwiches." Heat a large nonstick skillet or griddle over medium heat. Spray it with cooking spray and place the tortilla sandwiches on it. Allow them to cook until their bottoms begin to turn golden brown, then spray the top tortillas with oil and turn them. Continue cooking until the bottom tortillas begin to brown then place them on each of 4 serving plates.

Cook the eggs and finish the dish. Spray more cooking spray onto the skillet and cook the eggs, either up or over easy, or you may poach them. When they are done, place them on top of the tortilla "sandwiches" and top each with 2 tablespoons of the Romesco Sauce.

ANTOJITOS MEXICANOS

LITTLE MEXICAN WHIMS

LITTLE MEXICAN WHIMS could not be a more appropriate description of these simple tortilla- and corn-based foods, which include the likes of tacos, enchiladas, quesadillas, burritos, chimichangas, tostadas, and flautas and which have won the hearts of Americans and brought crowds of them to Mexican restaurants. Among other things, this branch of Mexican cooking provides the secret to the success of most Mexican restaurants in the United States, one you can easily use at home.

The secret is that almost all *antojitos* consist of three basic items: a filling, such as shredded chicken, fajitas, or simply refried beans; a wrap, usually a corn or flour tortilla; and a garnish, such as cheese, sour cream, guacamole, or salsa. Here's how it works. Assuming it already has tortillas and garnishes, if a restaurant prepares five fillings and uses those five fillings to make just the seven different items mentioned above, it will have thirty-five menu items. If it uses both flour and corn tortillas for some of the items, it will have even more. And if it serves some of the filling items, such as *carnitas* or fajitas, as entrées, there will be even more. All that for preparing just five fillings, some rice and beans, and a few salsas and sauces; grating some cheese; making some guacamole; and buying some tortillas!

You can use this secret at home to quickly produce anything from nutritious snacks to complete meals. For snacks, first lay in some tortillas. Next, make a couple of good salsas, including some pico de gallo, and have some cheese on hand and maybe an avocado for guacamole. Next, make and refrigerate one or more of your favorite fillings from the ones that follow or from other parts of the book. For example, you might choose one of the picadillos (ground meat fillings), fajita-style grilled chicken, Minilla de Pescado, or a vegetarian filling. If you make just one, you will be able to prepare almost any *antojito*, from tacos to burritos to tostadas, and do so very quickly because the fillings are easily heated in a microwave. For entrées, at half power, heat whatever filling you made and serve it with some salsa, rice, and/or beans, all of which also microwave well.

The recipes in this category are for fillings that can be used in many different *antojitos*. While they will also be featured in specific recipes for which they are particularly popular, they are listed here by themselves in hopes that readers will be inspired to create their own specialties.

Picadillo de los Turcos

TURKS' PICADILLO

14 servings, 1 taco per serving

PER SERVING | 90 calories | 6 g protein
9 g carbohydrates | 3.5 g total fat
(0.5 g saturated) | 15 mg cholesterol
1 g fiber | 6 g sugar | 190 mg sodium

This recipe delivers a lot of flavor for very little work. Spain, which was occupied by the Moors for hundreds of years, brought an important Middle Eastern influence to Mexican cooking. In Mexico the word turco *(Turk) often refers generically to things Middle Eastern. This filling makes a delicious change from the usual picadillos. It is perfect for* chiles rellenos, *but also works well in simpler fare, including soft tacos, tostadas, or flautas. To avoid having to buy different dried fruits, simply purchase a package of mixed fruit bits that includes apples, apricots, raisins, and pears.*

INGREDIENTS

1 tablespoon extra-virgin olive oil
½ cup chopped white onion, ¼-inch dice
1 large serrano chile, finely chopped, or substitute 1 jalapeño
2 cloves garlic, minced
¾ pound lean ground turkey (ideally, 3% fat)
¼ cup sliced black olives
1 (14½-ounce) can diced fire-roasted tomatoes
¼ cup chopped pecans
¾ cup finely chopped mixed dried fruit
½ teaspoon dried rubbed sage
1 teaspoon dried thyme
½ teaspoon dried marjoram
¾ teaspoon salt
¼ cup loosely packed chopped cilantro

DIRECTIONS

Heat a skillet over medium heat, add the oil, onions, and chile, and sauté until the onions are soft but not browned, 3–5 minutes. Add the garlic and cook another 30 seconds. Add the ground turkey and continue cooking, breaking it up with a large spoon, until the turkey has cooked through. Add the remaining ingredients and simmer until nearly all the moisture has evaporated, about 10 minutes.

Minilla
de Pescado

MINCED FISH FILLING

8 servings, 1 taco per serving

PER SERVING | 120 calories | 10 g protein
3 g carbohydrates | 7 g total fat
(1 g saturated) | 35 mg cholesterol
1 g fiber | 1 g sugar | 90 mg sodium

I adapted this recipe from one I found in Cocina jarocha *(Veracruz Cooking) by María Luisa Zamudio and Alida Gutiérrez Zamora. Besides being tasty, it is also easy to prepare and inexpensive. In Veracruz it is made with several types of fish, but I particularly like it made with farm-raised catfish. It can be served as an appetizer or snack with tortilla chips or used as a filling for Tacos de Minilla de Pescado (page 127). If you are eating it with chips, it is best served at room temperature, but for tacos it should be hot. You can make it in advance, refrigerate it, and then bring it to whatever temperature you want in a microwave.*

INGREDIENTS

3 cups water
½ cup dry sherry
2 cloves garlic, peeled and smashed
2 bay leaves
1 pound catfish fillets, or another mild fish
⅔ cup very finely chopped Roma tomatoes
¼ cup minced green olives
3 tablespoons minced pickled jalapeños, stems and seeds removed
2 tablespoons minced cilantro, divided
3 tablespoons extra-virgin olive oil
⅔ cup minced onions

DIRECTIONS

Make the poaching liquid. Put the water, sherry, garlic, and bay leaves in a medium-sized saucepan. Bring the mixture to a boil over high heat, boil for 1 minute, then remove from the heat.

Poach the fish. Add the fish to the poaching liquid and bring the liquid to a bare simmer. Poach until the fish is nearly cooked through, about 5 minutes. Remove the pan from the heat and leave the fish in the poaching liquid for 20 minutes.

Finish the recipe. Remove the fish from the pan and reserve 1 cup of the poaching liquid. Chop the fish very finely and put it into a bowl with the tomatoes, olives, jalapeños, and 1 tablespoon cilantro. Heat the oil in a skillet over medium heat, then add the onions and cook, stirring frequently, until they are soft but not browned, 3–4 minutes. Add the fish and the other ingredients, including the reserved poaching liquid. Bring to a low simmer and cook until all the liquid has evaporated, about 10 minutes.

Salmón Ahumado con Salsa de Aguacate y Trufas

SMOKED SALMON WITH
TRUFFLED AVOCADO SAUCE

10–12 servings, 1 taco per serving

PER SERVING | 130 calories | 12 g protein
3 g carbohydrates | 9 g total fat
(2 g saturated) | 30 mg cholesterol
2 g fiber | 0 g sugar | 260 mg sodium

This alta cocina recipe has many delicious and healthy uses, including as a salad (page 98) and a filling for tacos (page 128). It also makes a great sandwich filling. It is particularly good when paired with goat cheese and Mango Salsa and is an easy way to add more salmon to your diet with very little preparation. Look for smoked salmon that is thinly sliced and that has the least amount of salt, around 250 milligrams for each 2 ounces. The avocado portion of the recipe is also used as a sauce for scallops (page 201). A small amount of truffle oil adds an unexpected bit of sophistication and flavor to both dishes.

INGREDIENTS

2 large avocados, about 12 ounces fruit

2 tablespoons freshly squeezed lime juice

4 teaspoons good-quality white truffle oil

½ teaspoon salt

5 tablespoons sour cream or Tofutti

1 tablespoon minced serrano chile

4 tablespoons finely chopped cilantro

8 ounces thinly sliced smoked salmon, chopped
    into roughly ½-inch squares

DIRECTIONS

Make the sauce. Put all the ingredients except the salmon in the bowl of a food processor and process for 2 minutes, or until smooth and glistening.
    Complete the filling. Spoon the sauce into a bowl and stir in the salmon.

Carne de Puerco al Pastor

SHEPHERD'S-STYLE
PORK FILLING

10 servings, 1 taco per serving

PER SERVING | 90 calories | 14 g protein
2 g carbohydrates | 2.5 g total fat
(0.5 g saturated) | 45 mg cholesterol
0 g fiber | 1 g sugar | 190 mg sodium

This recipe is a slimming, healthful, and delicious version of the traditional pork filling that is cooked on vertical spits in street stalls all over Mexico and used to make tacos al pastor *(shepherd's tacos). In northern Mexico they are often called* tacos de trompo *(top tacos) because the meat on the spit resembles a spinning top. While you can't match the taste of slow-roasted fatty pork shoulder, I do not hesitate to offer this recipe as a separate but equal alternative. Made with very lean pork tenderloin and soaked in a fabulous version of the traditional marinade, the result is both tender and very satisfying, but it must be grilled over very high heat until the meat hits medium-rare. By the time you serve it, it should be medium, with no pink.*

¾ **cup orange juice**

¼ **cup pineapple juice**

3 **guajillo chiles, toasted and rehydrated** (pages 15–16)

¾ **teaspoon cinnamon, preferably** *canela*

2 **cloves garlic, roughly chopped**

½ **tablespoon agave nectar or honey**

1 **teaspoon salt**

½ **teaspoon black pepper**

1 **tablespoon vegetable oil**

1½ **pounds pork tenderloin, cut lengthwise into ½-inch-thick slices**

DIRECTIONS

Make the marinade. Bring the juices to a boil in a small saucepan and continue boiling until they are reduced to ½ cup. Remove the pan from the heat.

Drain and discard the water from the rehydrated chiles. Put the chiles in a blender, add the reduced juices, cinnamon, garlic, agave nectar, salt, and pepper and purée. Pour the marinade into a large bowl, and stir in the vegetable oil and the meat. Marinate, refrigerated, for 3 hours.

Grill and chop the meat. Heat a charcoal grill or a gas grill as hot as you can. Grill the meat until it is medium-rare. If the fire is hot enough, the meat will be slightly charred on both sides and continue to cook. Chop the meat into bite-sized pieces for tacos and other *antojitos*, or serve as is.

Picadillo de Carne de Res

BEEF FILLING

8 servings

PER SERVING | 100 calories | 13 g protein
5 g carbohydrates | 3 g total fat
(1.5 g saturated) | 35 mg cholesterol
0 g fiber | 1 g sugar | 210 mg sodium

Picadillos, or ground meat fillings, are much more popular in the United States than in Mexico, where shredded meat is much more common. This Tex-Mex version is easy to make, tasty, and, for a beef filling, low in fat and calories. It is made by simmering very lean ground meat until tender and flavorful, with potatoes, Chile Sauce or salsa, and spices. The potatoes add a nice texture and flavor but can be omitted to reduce carbs. While the recipe calls for my homemade Chile Sauce and canned tomato sauce, you could substitute any tomato-based salsa for both ingredients, either purchased (be aware of the sodium content) or made at home. ▶▶

1 pound 96% lean ground beef

2½ cups water

½ cup Chile Sauce (page 45), preferably made with ancho chiles

⅓ cup tomato sauce

¾ cup finely chopped peeled russet potatoes

¾ teaspoon ground cumin

1 teaspoon dried leaf oregano

1 teaspoon rice vinegar

¼ heaping teaspoon salt, or to taste

DIRECTIONS

Bring to a boil and skim the picadillo. Place the meat in a medium-sized pot, add the water, and stir to dissolve the meat into a slurry. Bring to a boil and lower the heat to a simmer. As the beef simmers, a thick brown liquid will bubble to the top. Skim it off with a slotted spoon and discard it.

Finish the picadillo. Stir in the remaining ingredients and cook at a low simmer until all the liquid has evaporated, 35–40 minutes. Turn the heat to very low and continue cooking until you cannot see any more liquid, 5–10 minutes.

Carne Seca

DRIED MEAT

About 12 taco filling portions

PER SERVING | 170 calories | 13 g protein 2 g carbohydrates | 12 g total fat (3.5 g saturated) | 30 mg cholesterol 0 g fiber | 1 g sugar | 130 mg sodium

The name may not sound exciting, but this is my favorite filling. I fell in love with it at Tucson's El Charro Café, one of the oldest and best Mexican restaurants in the United States. The filling is the best I have ever found for burritos and chimichangas, and is also terrific in tacos, quesadillas, and tortas, and as the main ingredient in Beef Salpicón (page 101). El Charro air-dries its beef in a screened cage on top of the restaurant. For those of us who live in less sunny, more humid climates, El Charro's owner, Carlotta Dunn Flores, provides instructions in her cookbook, and the following is my take on her recipe. One ingredient she uses, garlic purée, is a terrific way to add garlic to everything from soups to beans and rice. In this version I use flank steak because it is so lean and shreds easily. The broth created by braising the meat is perfect for soups or enchilada sauce, so just strain and freeze it.

INGREDIENTS

2 tablespoons canola oil

2 pounds flank steak

2 (½-inch) slices onion

10 cloves garlic, 2 of them smashed and the others coarsely chopped

½ teaspoon dried leaf oregano

2 tablespoons freshly squeezed lime juice

½ cup water

¼ cup extra-virgin olive oil

⅓ cup minced white onion

½ cup roasted, peeled, and chopped poblano chile (page 16)

¾ cup chopped fresh tomato

½ teaspoon salt

½ teaspoon black pepper

DIRECTIONS

Preheat your oven to 300°F.

Braise the meat. Heat a Dutch oven or similar oven-safe pot over medium-high heat, add the oil, and sear the meat on both sides until brown and crusty, about 1 minute per side. You will probably have 2 pieces of steak, so sear them one at a time. Pour off any excess oil and add enough water to just cover the meat. Bring to a boil, skim any thick brown liquid that rises to the surface, and add the onion slices, 2 garlic cloves, and oregano. Cover and bake for 2½ hours.

Shred the meat. Remove the pot from the oven and remove the meat to a plate to cool for a few minutes. You can shred it by hand, with your fingers or with two forks, but a much easier way is to cut the meat into 2-inch pieces and shred it in 2 or 3 batches in a food processor fitted with the short dough blade (the regular chopping blade will cut the meat too finely). You should end up with about 4 cups shredded beef, weighing about 1 pound.

Make the garlic purée and dry the meat. Raise the oven temperature to 325°F. Blend the remaining 8 cloves garlic with the water until completely puréed; spoon off and discard the foam. Toss the shredded beef with 2 tablespoons of the garlic purée and the lime juice and spread on a baking sheet. Bake, stirring every 5 minutes, until the beef is dry and crispy, 25–40 minutes.

Finish the filling. This is where the recipe really pops! Heat a 12-inch skillet over medium heat and add the olive oil and onions. Cook, stirring often, until the onions are soft but not browned, about 3 minutes. Add the poblano chile, tomato, dried meat, salt, pepper, and 2 more tablespoons garlic purée. Cook the meat, stirring and turning it nearly constantly, for 3–5 minutes.

Carne Guisada

STEWED BEEF

4 entrée servings, or about 10 tacos

PER SERVING | 130 calories | 13 g protein
4 g carbohydrates | 7 g total fat
(1.5 g saturated) | 35 mg cholesterol
1 g fiber | 1 g sugar | 125 mg sodium

This classic Tex-Mex beef stew is a perfect example of the less-is-more principle of Mexican cooking and particularly of the Tex-Mex variety. So focused were early cooks on producing economical meals that dishes like this one are actually best when made with small amounts of inexpensive ingredients. It is particularly good in flour tortilla tacos and burritos.

INGREDIENTS

3 tablespoons canola oil
1¼ pounds eye of round or a similarly lean cut of beef,
    cut into ½-inch pieces
⅔ cup finely chopped white onion
2 tablespoons chopped jalapeño pepper
½ cup chopped green bell pepper
¾ cup chopped tomato
2 teaspoons granulated garlic
½ slightly heaping teaspoon ground cumin
2 tablespoons canned tomato purée
¼ heaping teaspoon salt, or to taste
¼ teaspoon black pepper
2 tablespoons all-purpose flour

DIRECTIONS

Sear the meat. Heat a medium-sized pot or Dutch oven over medium-high to high heat. Add 1½ tablespoons of the oil and the meat and cook until the meat is browned on one side, about 30 seconds. Stir until it is slightly browned on all sides. Remove the meat and reserve.

Soften the vegetables. Lower the heat to medium and add the onion, jalapeño, and bell pepper to the pot. Cook, stirring frequently, until they are soft but not browned, 3–4 minutes. Add the tomato and cook 1 minute.

Make the stew. Return the browned meat to the pot and add enough hot tap water to cover it by about 1 inch. Add the granulated garlic, cumin, tomato purée, salt, and pepper and bring to a boil. Lower the heat to a medium simmer, cover the pot, and cook for 2 hours. Check the pot frequently, especially toward the end, to make sure that all the liquid has not evaporated. At the end of 2 hours there should be enough liquid to come about halfway up the other ingredients, and it should be fairly thick. It you are left with too much liquid, simply remove the top and cook at a fast simmer until enough evaporates. If there is too little liquid, add a little more water.

Make the roux and finish the stew. While the stew is cooking, heat a small saucepan over medium-low heat or just a little lower. Add the remaining 1½ tablespoons oil. Whisk in the flour and cook, whisking constantly, until the roux is a light brown color, 3–4 minutes. When the liquid in the stew is at the right level and consistency, stir in 1 teaspoon of the roux and continue cooking for about 45 seconds. If necessary, keep adding roux, a little at a time, until the liquid is thick enough to coat the back of the spoon and the stew holds together. This usually requires no more than 1 or 2 teaspoons of roux.

Chorizo

10 servings, about 2 ounces each

PER SERVING | 200 calories
10 g protein | 2 g carbohydrates
5 g total fat (1 g saturated)
30 mg cholesterol | 0 g fiber
2 g sugar | 400 mg sodium

Unlike Spanish chorizo, which is usually cooked in its casing, most Mexican chorizo is really bulk sausage that is removed from its wrapping before cooking. Like most sausages, chorizo obtains much of its flavor and appeal from fat, and there is not much you can do about that to create anything close to an ideal nutrition profile. Experience has taught me that with every bit of fat that is removed, a certain amount of flavor and mouthfeel also vanishes. However, I have also found that, while it is important to keep most of the fat content, much of it can be replaced with healthier fat, such as extra-virgin olive oil. While that reduces the succulent flavor of pork fat, it is also much better than nothing for those who want to reduce saturated fat in their diet.

INGREDIENTS

1 pound pork tenderloin, cut into ½-inch pieces
2½ tablespoons pure ancho or mild New Mexico chile powder
3 cloves garlic, very finely chopped or put through a garlic press
¼ teaspoon ground cloves
½ teaspoon cinnamon, preferably *canela*
½ teaspoon dried leaf oregano
½ teaspoon dried marjoram
½ teaspoon dried thyme
1¼ teaspoons salt
1 tablespoon plus 2 teaspoons cider vinegar
1 tablespoon plus 2 teaspoons rice vinegar
⅓ cup extra-virgin olive oil, plus more for frying

DIRECTIONS

Partially freeze the meat. Put the cut-up pork in a bowl or on a plate and put it in the freezer until it is partially frozen, about a half hour. Stir it every 10 minutes to keep it from sticking to the container.

Grind and flavor the chorizo. You can use a meat grinder or food processor. If using a meat grinder, put the partially frozen meat through the fine blade then mix it by hand with the remaining ingredients. If using a food processor, put the partially frozen meat in the bowl, add the remaining ingredients, and pulse using the steel blade until the meat is finely ground, ten to fifteen 1-second pulses; do not allow it to turn into a paste.

Cook the chorizo. Coat a skillet with a little extra-virgin olive oil and fry the chorizo over medium heat until it is cooked through and as crispy as you like.

Chorizo, Potatoes, and Carrots

8 servings, about 2 ounces each, as a filling for antojitos.

PER SERVING | 120 calories | 6 g protein 11 g carbohydrates | 5 g total fat (1 g saturated) | 15 mg cholesterol 1 g fiber | 2 g sugar | 210 mg sodium

Chorizo has a natural affinity to potatoes and carrots as attested by the Tacos Potosinos recipe (page 129), and that combination makes a popular filling, especially for tacos and quesadillas. It also makes for great breakfast tacos when combined with scrambled eggs.

INGREDIENTS

2½ cups peeled and diced potatoes, ¼-inch dice
1 cup peeled and diced carrots, ¼-inch dice
1½ tablespoons extra-virgin olive oil
8 ounces Chorizo (page 119)
3 tablespoons finely chopped cilantro

DIRECTIONS

Parboil the potatoes and carrots. Place the potatoes and carrots in a saucepan and add enough water to cover by one inch. Cook until the vegetables just begin to soften. Pour them into a strainer and discard the water.

Fry the potatoes and carrots and finish the filling. Heat a skillet over medium-high heat, add the olive oil, potatoes, and carrots, and cook, stirring frequently, until the vegetables are soft on the inside and crispy and brown on the outside. Lower the heat to medium, add the Chorizo, and cook, breaking the meat up, until it is cooked through. Add the cilantro and serve.

Relleno de Hongos

MUSHROOM FILLING

Enough to fill about 8 large flour tortilla quesadillas or tacos, or 4 side dish servings. Nutrition calculations are for the quesadillas or tacos.

PER SERVING | 80 calories | 3 g protein 5 g carbohydrates | 6 g total fat (1 g saturated) | 0 mg cholesterol 1 g fiber | 2 g sugar | 150 mg sodium

This recipe makes a delicious vegetarian filling for antojitos that can also be used as a side dish, especially with broiled meats and poultry. I especially like it with Quesadillas (page 145). It is also terrific as part of a vegetarian entrée, perhaps combined with the Spinach Filling (page 121). It can be made entirely with common button mushrooms, but the more exotic mushrooms you add, the more complex and interesting the dish will be. I often combine the mushrooms with the Caramelized Rajas recipe (page 70) for a great filling or a topping for grilled meats or poultry.

INGREDIENTS

1½ pounds mushrooms, chopped into ½-inch pieces
3½ tablespoons extra-virgin olive oil
⅓ cup finely chopped shallots
3 tablespoons minced, stemmed, and seeded jalapeño pepper
3 cloves finely chopped garlic
1 teaspoon dried leaf oregano
½ teaspoon salt
Black pepper, to taste
1 teaspoon dried tarragon

3 tablespoons finely chopped fresh chives

2 tablespoons finely chopped fresh parsley

DIRECTIONS

Preheat your oven to 400°F.

Roast the mushrooms. In a bowl, toss the mushrooms with 2 tablespoons of the olive oil, spread them onto a baking sheet, and roast them for 10 minutes. Remove the sheet from the oven and put it on the stove top, tilted to allow the juices to accumulate away from the mushrooms while they cool. When the mushrooms have cooled, collect the juice and reserve it and the mushrooms separately.

Finish the mushrooms. In a large skillet, heat the remaining 1½ tablespoons olive oil over medium-high heat. Add the shallots and jalapeño and sauté until they begin to soften, about 2 minutes. Add the garlic and continue cooking until it has cooked through but not browned, 30–45 seconds. Add the mushrooms and the remaining ingredients except the mushroom juice and sauté until the mushrooms begin to brown. Add the mushroom juice and continue cooking and stirring until it has evaporated, 1–2 minutes.

Spinach Filling

Enough for about 11 large flour tortilla quesadillas, or 6 side dish servings. Nutrition calculations are for the quesadillas.

PER SERVING | 120 calories | 7 g protein
5 g carbohydrates | 8 g total fat
(3.5 g saturated) | 15 mg cholesterol
2 g fiber | 1 g sugar | 340 mg sodium

This vegetarian filling is delicious with quesadillas, which are easy to prepare since the cheese is already in the filling. The filling also heats up nicely in a microwave and makes a great accompaniment for poultry, a delicious filling for enchiladas, and a tasty topping for nachos. Be sure to squeeze the thawed spinach in a towel to remove as much of the liquid as possible or the filling will be watery. One of my favorite dinners is to combine this dish with the mushroom filling for a great vegetarian meal.

INGREDIENTS

¼ cup plus 2 tablespoons 30% lower-fat cream cheese, room temperature

2 tablespoons room-temperature sour cream

6 ounces part skim milk mozzarella, grated

1 tablespoon extra-virgin olive oil

1 tablespoon minced serrano chile

½ cup pitted, coarsely chopped black olives

4 cloves garlic, peeled and minced or put through a garlic press

2 (10-ounce) packages frozen leaf spinach, thawed, coarsely chopped, and squeezed dry

½ teaspoon salt

1½ tablespoons freshly squeezed lime juice

¼ cup chopped toasted pecans ▶▶

DIRECTIONS

Combine the dairy products. In a food processor or by hand, thoroughly combine the cream cheese, sour cream, and mozzarella and reserve.

Sauté the spinach and remaining ingredients. Heat the olive oil in a large skillet over medium heat. Add the chile and olives and stir-fry for about 1 minute. Add the garlic and stir-fry for another 30 seconds. Stir in the spinach and salt and continue cooking for about 2 minutes. Stir in the lime juice and cook 1 minute. Remove the skillet from the heat and allow the spinach to cool enough so that it will not melt the cheese when they are combined.

Finish the dish. When the spinach mixture has cooled, stir it and the pecans into the dairy mixture until well combined.

PLAIN & SPICY SHREDDED CHICKEN OR TURKEY

Many cooks in both homes and restaurants use a plain shredded chicken filling for *antojitos*, while others prefer one that is spicier. In some places, such as Baja California, turkey is used in place of chicken, a choice that can be less expensive and just as good or better. The following recipe provides instructions for both plain and spicy alternatives. The latter is particularly good with burritos and flour tacos.

Plain Shredded Chicken or Turkey

About 8 two-ounce portions

PER SERVING | 60 calories | 12 g protein 0 g carbohydrates | 1.5 g total fat (0 g saturated) | 35 mg cholesterol 0 g fiber | 0 g sugar | 210 mg sodium

INGREDIENTS

1 pound boneless, skinless chicken or turkey breasts, cut into 2-inch pieces
6 cups water
½ teaspoon salt

DIRECTIONS

Put the chicken or turkey in a pot, cover it with 6 cups water, bring it to a boil, and simmer until it is cooked through, 10–15 minutes. Remove the meat and reserve the cooking liquid to use in the Spicy Shredded Chicken or Turkey. Shred the meat, stir in the salt, and you are finished.

Spicy Shredded Chicken or Turkey

4 servings, about 8 tacos or 4 burritos

PER SERVING | 90 calories | 13 g protein 7 g carbohydrates | 1.5 g total fat (0 g saturated) | 35 mg cholesterol 2 g fiber | 3 g sugar | 230 mg sodium

If you want the spicy and more flavorful version, reserve the shredded poultry and cooking liquid from the Plain Shredded Chicken or Turkey, leave out the salt, and proceed.

INGREDIENTS

1 tablespoon extra-virgin olive oil
1 cup sliced white onion
3 tablespoons finely chopped jalapeño pepper
1 cup chopped green bell pepper
4 garlic cloves, finely chopped
¾ cup chopped tomato
1 recipe Plain Shredded Chicken or Turkey (page 122)
½ tablespoon chopped canned chipotle chile
½ teaspoon ground cumin
1½ teaspoons dried leaf oregano
1 cup tomato sauce, no salt added, if possible
Reserved cooking liquid from Plain Shredded Chicken or Turkey
2 bay leaves
¼ cup chopped cilantro

DIRECTIONS

Make the spicy filling. Heat the olive oil in a pot or Dutch oven over medium heat. Add the onion, jalapeño, bell pepper, and garlic and cook, stirring frequently, until the onion and pepper are just soft, 3–4 minutes. Add the tomatoes and cook another minute. Stir in the reserved Plain Shredded Chicken or Turkey and the chipotle, cumin, oregano, and tomato sauce. Add the reserved cooking liquid from the Plain Shredded Chicken or Turkey and the bay leaves, bring to a boil, reduce the heat to low, and cook at a low to medium simmer until there is just a little liquid left in the pot. This can take anywhere from a half hour to a little over an hour, depending on the heat. Stir in the cilantro and continue cooking until nearly all the liquid is gone.

Huitlacoche and Mushroom Filling

Enough filling for about 8 quesadillas, 20 medium-sized stuffed mushrooms, or 4 large portobello mushroom entrées

PER SERVING | 120 calories | 5 g protein
5 g carbohydrates | 9 g total fat
(2.5 g saturated) | 10 mg cholesterol
1 g fiber | 2 g sugar | 250 mg sodium

Huitlacoche is the relatively unknown and even less frequently sampled corn fungi (page 12) that are esteemed as a delicacy in Mexico. While huitlacoche can be a bit assertive, fortunately, it pairs beautifully with milder flavored mushrooms and cheese. This filling has many potential uses, but my favorites are in quesadillas and stuffed mushrooms, either small ones for appetizers or large ones for a vegetarian entrée. Vegans may eliminate the sour cream and cheese and use oil in place of the butter substitute. The dish heats up well in an oven or microwave.

INGREDIENTS

1 pound mushrooms, chopped into ½-inch pieces
4 teaspoons extra-virgin olive oil
2 tablespoons butter substitute
¼ cup finely chopped shallots
3 cloves garlic, finely chopped
⅓ cup chopped tomato
½ cup chopped roasted, peeled, and seeded poblano pepper (page 16)
1 (7-ounce) can huitlacoche (page 12)
½ teaspoon dried leaf oregano
½ teaspoon kosher salt
¼ teaspoon black pepper
1 sprig epazote (optional)
2 tablespoons brandy
3 tablespoons finely chopped fresh chives
2 tablespoons finely chopped fresh parsley
3 tablespoons sour cream
3 ounces part skim milk mozzarella, grated

DIRECTIONS

Preheat your oven to 400°F.

Roast the mushrooms. Toss the mushrooms with the olive oil, spread them onto a baking sheet, and roast them for 10 minutes. Remove the baking sheet from the oven and place on the stove top, tilted to allow the juices to accumulate away from the mushrooms while they cool. When they have cooled, reserve the mushrooms and discard the juice.

Sauté and finish the mushrooms. In a 12-inch skillet, melt the butter substitute over between medium and medium-high heat. Add the shallots and garlic and sauté until they are almost soft, about 2 minutes. Add the tomato and poblano pepper and sauté an additional minute or two. Stir in the reserved mushrooms, huitlacoche, oregano, salt, pepper, and epazote, if using.

Scrape some of the ingredients to the side of the pan, leaving about 3 inches in the center. Pour the brandy into that space and immediately light it with a long-handled fire starter or similar safe implement. When the brandy flames, shake the pan and stir the mushroom mixture into the brandy. Stir in the chives, parsley, and sour cream and cook 1 more minute. If you plan to use the filling immediately, stir in the cheese and remove the pan from the heat. If you will be using it later, allow the filling to cool enough so that it will not melt the cheese and then add it. Refrigerate until ready to use.

TACOS

Tacos are undoubtedly Mexico's best known and most popular food. While they are made with both corn and flour tortillas, because of their lower fat and calories and the nutritional value of nixtamalized corn, corn tortillas are generally considered to be the best choice for the health conscious. But the recipe for Low-Fat Flour Tortillas (page 32) does make them a reasonable option. Making crispy, low-fat taco shells that don't come with the extra calories and fat of deep-frying is difficult, but the truth is that in Mexico they are not served very often. Much more common are soft tacos or those made with lightly fried, semicrisp shells that are easy to fold and do not break at the first bite, dumping the filling into your lap.

For a low-fat version of the semicrisp variety, heat a nonstick skillet over medium-high heat and spray it with cooking spray. Spray both sides of a corn tortilla and cook it, turning frequently, until it begins to brown and crisp. Another option is to bake the oil-sprayed tortillas in a 350°F oven for about 4 minutes, or until they just begin to crisp.

For truly low-fat soft tacos, you can heat corn tortillas in a microwave with no loss of quality. You can also do this with flour tortillas, but you must do it very carefully, as just a few seconds too long will cause the tortilla to become rubbery. It is much better to take the small amount of extra time to reheat them on a skillet or griddle over medium heat.

My favorite way of serving tacos is family-style, where the filling, tortillas, salsas, guacamole, etc., are placed on the table, and diners help themselves.

Tex-Mex Tacos

4 servings, 2 tacos each

PER SERVING | 360 calories
21 g protein | 37 g carbohydrates
15 g total fat (6 g saturated)
20 mg cholesterol | 7 g fiber
5 g sugar | 640 mg sodium

My favorite Tex-Mex tacos are made with semicrisp rather than crisp corn tortilla shells. They are easier to work with, and I think they are just as good. I prefer frying the shells in about 1 inch of oil in a skillet as opposed to baking them in the oven, but I often do the latter because then each shell has about 80 fewer calories.

To bake the shells, preheat your oven to 350°F. Spray the tortillas on both sides with a little cooking spray and lay them directly on the oven rack. Bake for about 4 minutes, or until they are just beginning to stiffen. Take them out of the oven, allow them to cool until you can handle them, and fold them in half.

Alternatively, you may make the tacos with hot flour tortillas. ▶▶

8 corn tortilla taco shells (prepared as described above)
   or hot flour tortillas
½ cup Refried Beans (page 67)
½ cup Guacamole (page 59)
½ recipe Beef Picadillo, about 8 ounces (page 115)
2 cups shredded iceberg lettuce
1 cup chopped tomato
4 ounces part skim milk mozzarella, grated
3 tablespoons grated *cotija* cheese
Salsa

DIRECTIONS

Make the tacos. Spread about 2 tablespoons Refried Beans on half of each taco shell or flour tortilla. Spread about 2 tablespoons Guacamole on the other half. Spread about 2 ounces Picadillo between the beans and guacamole and top with the lettuce, tomato, cheeses, and salsa.

Turks' Picadillo Tacos

SOFT TACOS WITH A SAVORY GROUND TURKEY FILLING

4 servings, 2 tacos each

PER SERVING | 360 calories
17 g protein | 38 g carbohydrates
16 g total fat (6 g saturated)
55 mg cholesterol | 5 g fiber
11 g sugar | 530 mg sodium

Because everything can be prepared well ahead and because they come together so quickly, these tacos are a good choice for anything from lunch to a mid-afternoon snack or a weeknight dinner. Once the filling is in the fridge, the tacos can literally be made on a whim and with very little effort. Pepper Jack cheese is specified because it goes so well with the filling, but ordinary Monterey Jack, mozzarella, mild cheddar, Oaxaca, provolone, and goat cheese also work well. The recipe makes enough for about 8 tacos. If you are making fewer than that, just refrigerate the remaining filling to be used later.

INGREDIENTS

1 pound Turks' Picadillo (page 112)
8 corn tortillas
4 ounces pepper Jack cheese, grated
Your favorite salsa(s)

DIRECTIONS

The Turks' Picadillo should be hot enough that the cheese will begin to melt on contact. If you need to reheat it, do so in a microwave. Heat the tortillas in a tortilla warmer or wrapped in a towel in a microwave.

To serve family-style, place all the ingredients on the table. Spoon about 2 ounces of the filling on a tortilla, sprinkle on some cheese, drizzle on some salsa, and enjoy!

Tacos de Minilla de Pescado

TACOS WITH MINCED FISH FILLING

4 servings, 2 tacos each

PER SERVING | 370 calories
20 g protein | 29 g carbohydrates
20 g total fat (3 g saturated)
60 mg cholesterol | 5 g fiber
4 g sugar | 320 mg sodium

With the current popularity of fish tacos, I am surprised not to have seen this dish from Veracruz served in the United States. It is delicious and easy to prepare in advance and is both good for you and inexpensive. If you do make it ahead of time, just reheat it in a microwave.

INGREDIENTS

1 recipe Minilla de Pescado (page 113)
1 recipe Guacamole (page 59)
8 hot corn tortillas
Salsa(s)
Lime wedges

DIRECTIONS

Place all the ingredients on the table and allow diners to make their own soft tacos.

Tacos Tropicales

TROPICAL SALMON TACOS

4 servings, 2 tacos each

PER SERVING | 410 calories | 30 g protein
50 g carbohydrates | 10 g total fat
(1 g saturated) | 65 mg cholesterol
7 g fiber | 6 g sugar | 85 mg sodium

While salmon is not indigenous to Mexico, it is nevertheless popular and goes very well with the famous Yucatán seasoning paste called achiote. Carried by most Hispanic groceries, achiote comes in small cardboard packages and is very inexpensive. Adding a small amount of the adobo rub used in the recipe for Salmon Escabeche with Avocado-Mango Salsa (pages 194–195) to the paste is not essential but does improve the dish. In addition to a filling for tacos, the salmon can also be served whole as an entrée. These tacos are made with two overlapped corn tortillas.

INGREDIENTS

2 tablespoons packaged achiote paste (about 1 ounce)
1 teaspoon adobo rub from the recipe for Salmon Escabeche
    (optional, page 195)
4–5 teaspoons orange juice
1 pound salmon fillets, skins removed
8 corn tortillas
½ cup Jalisco-style Pico de Gallo (page 38)
½ cup finely shredded cabbage
Your favorite salsa

DIRECTIONS

Marinate the salmon. Mix the achiote, adobo rub, and orange juice into a paste and spread it on one side of the salmon. Marinate for at least 4 hours or overnight in the refrigerator. ▸▸

Grill the salmon. Heat a charcoal or gas grill to medium-high or a grill pan over medium-high heat. Grill the salmon until it is just done but not overcooked, and chop it into bite-sized pieces.

Make the tacos. Heat the tortillas and place one on each of four plates. Lay another tortilla on the first one, 1–1½ inches off center. Put a line of chopped salmon lengthwise on the tortillas, top with Pico de Gallo, shredded cabbage, and salsa, and serve.

Tacos de Salmón Ahumado

SMOKED SALMON TACOS

6 servings, 2 tacos each

PER SERVING | 370 calories
28 g protein | 17 g carbohydrates
24 g total fat (7 g saturated)
75 mg cholesterol | 5 g fiber
6 g sugar | 680 mg sodium

These tacos combine the filling for Smoked Salmon with Truffled Avocado Sauce (page 114) with goat cheese and Mango Salsa (page 40) to create delicious soft tacos. They can be made with full-sized corn tortillas to make regular tacos or with small tortillas to be served as canapés.

INGREDIENTS

For the dressing
½ tablespoon sherry vinegar
⅛ teaspoon salt
⅛ teaspoon black pepper
2 tablespoons extra-virgin olive oil
3 ounces fresh spinach leaves

For the tacos
12 hot corn tortillas
1 recipe Smoked Salmon with Truffled Avocado Sauce (page 114)
4 ounces goat cheese
1 recipe Mango Salsa (page 40)

DIRECTIONS

Make the garnish. Whisk the vinegar in a medium-sized bowl with the salt and pepper. Gradually whisk in the olive oil. Add the spinach leaves, toss, and reserve.

Make the tacos. Spoon some of the smoked salmon mixture on half of a tortilla. Add some of the cheese, Mango Salsa, and the reserved garnish. Fold the taco in half and serve. Alternatively, the tacos may be served family-style.

Tacos Potosinos

POTOSÍ-STYLE TACOS

4 servings, 2 tacos each

PER SERVING | 350 calories
14 g protein | 47 g carbohydrates
12 g total fat (4 g saturated)
25 mg cholesterol | 6 g fiber
6 g sugar | 450 mg sodium

I fell in love with this dish the first time I tried it in the city of San Luis Potosí. More like enchiladas than tacos, they are a terrific example of a dish that is earthy, delicious, and naturally good for you. The traditional way to soften the tortillas is to dip them in Chile Sauce and fry them briefly in hot oil, which is awkward and messy. The technique I have developed does a fine job of imitating that process with much less effort and mess.

INGREDIENTS

For the vegetables
1 cup peeled, diced carrots, ¼–½-inch pieces, about 5 ounces
2 cups peeled, diced potatoes, ¼–½-inch pieces, about 10 ounces

For the tacos
½ cup Chile Sauce (page 45)
8 corn tortillas
Cooking spray
8 ounces *panela* cheese, grated
1 tablespoon extra-virgin olive oil
2 ounces Chorizo (page 119)
Reserved carrots and potatoes
¼ teaspoon salt
4 cups shredded iceberg lettuce

DIRECTIONS

Prepare the vegetables. Cook the carrots in simmering water until they are just tender. Using a slotted spoon, transfer them to a strainer and rinse under cold running water to stop the cooking. Cook and cool the potatoes in the same manner.

Prepare the tortillas. Place the tortillas on a work surface, brush one side with Chile Sauce, and spray with cooking spray. Turn the tortillas over and repeat. Wrap the tortillas in a kitchen towel or put them in a microwave-safe tortilla warmer and microwave on High for about 35 seconds, or until they are very soft.

Make the tacos. Put about ¾ of an ounce of cheese just off center on a softened tortilla and roll it as you would an enchilada. Repeat with the remaining tortillas, using about ¾ of the cheese in all and reserving the rest for the garnish. Place the rolled tacos on a large plate.

Heat a large skillet over medium heat. Add the oil and Chorizo and cook, breaking up the Chorizo with a spoon, until it is cooked through, about 2 minutes. Add the reserved carrots and potatoes and the salt and raise the heat to medium-high. Fry, stirring almost constantly, until the potatoes just begin to brown. ▸▸

Just before serving, make a small bed of lettuce on each of four plates, reserving a little for garnish. Brush more Chile Sauce on the tacos and heat them in a microwave until just warm, about 40 seconds. Place 2 tacos on each plate and top with the vegetables and Chorizo. Top with more lettuce and the reserved cheese.

Tacos Árabes

ARAB TACOS

4 servings

PER SERVING | 470 calories
36 g protein | 41 g carbohydrates
17 g total fat (3.5 g saturated)
90 mg cholesterol | 6 g fiber
3 g sugar | 310 mg sodium

Tacos Árabes are a specialty of the city of Puebla. They are served with Pan Árabe, an Arab bread that resembles a cross between a flour tortilla and pita bread. I was surprised that the filling is made from pork until I learned that most of the early Middle Eastern immigrants to Mexico were Lebanese Christians rather than Muslims. The meat is cooked on vertical skewers, much like that for Tacos al Pastor, except a different marinade is used. On my last visit to Puebla I found what has become my favorite version of the dish in a small café. The marinade was based on yogurt, with distinctively Middle Eastern seasonings. After several tries, I adapted a recipe from Saveur *magazine that accurately mimics that marinade, as does the use of flour tortillas made partially with whole wheat flour, as suggested in the section on tortillas as a stand-in for Pan Árabe. The dish is equally delicious with the traditional pork or with boneless, skinless chicken breast, and either goes well with the Grilled Rajas.*

INGREDIENTS

For the marinade
3 tablespoons extra-virgin olive oil
2 cups chopped white onion
¼ cup plain yogurt
¼ teaspoon ground ginger
2 cloves garlic, chopped
¼ teaspoon black pepper
½ teaspoon salt
¼ teaspoon cayenne
1 teaspoon ground coriander
¼ teaspoon ground nutmeg
⅛ teaspoon ground mace
½ teaspoon dried leaf oregano

For the tacos
Reserved marinade
1¼ pounds pork tenderloin, cut lengthwise into ½-inch slices, or boneless, skinless chicken breast, cut or pounded to ½-inch thickness
1 large avocado, sliced
Grilled Rajas (page 71)

Salsa

8 pieces hot Pan Árabe–style flour tortillas (page 32) or pita bread

DIRECTIONS

Make the marinade. Heat a skillet over medium heat, add the olive oil, and sauté 1 cup of the onions, stirring them frequently, until they are golden brown, turning down the heat as necessary to keep them from scorching. Reserve.

Put the cooked onions, raw onions, yogurt, ginger, garlic, pepper, salt, cayenne, coriander, nutmeg, mace, and oregano in a blender and purée.

Marinate the pork or chicken. Toss the pork or chicken with the marinade in a bowl and refrigerate for at least 6 hours or overnight.

Grill the pork or chicken. Prepare a wood or charcoal fire or heat a gas grill to very hot. Grill the pork or chicken until just cooked through and cut it into bite-sized pieces.

Prepare the tacos. Serve family-style by placing the pork or chicken, avocado slices, Rajas, salsa, and bread on the table so everyone can make their own tacos.

Tacos de Carne Asada

GRILLED STEAK TACOS

4 servings, 2 tacos each

PER SERVING | 430 calories | 31 g protein
39 g carbohydrates | 16 g total fat
(4 g saturated) | 75 mg cholesterol
5 g fiber | 3 g sugar | 560 mg sodium

These northern Mexican tacos are close to being my all-time favorite. Often made with skirt steak, they are just as good and a bit more tender when made using the Grilled Top Sirloin recipe. Like so many other antojitos, *they are easily made with already prepared and reheated ingredients, including the steak, and that is how the directions are written.*

INGREDIENTS

8 flour tortillas
½ cup Grilled Rajas (page 71)
1 pound Grilled Top Sirloin (page 174), cut into ½-inch pieces
Guacamole made from 1 large avocado (page 59)
Salsa

DIRECTIONS

Heat the tortillas. Warm the tortillas on a griddle or in a skillet and wrap them in a towel or put them into a tortilla warmer.

Heat the meat and rajas. If not making them from scratch, mix the Grilled Rajas and Grilled Top Sirloin in a microwave-safe dish and microwave at half power until they are hot, 45 seconds–1 minute.

To serve. Put the heated tortillas, meat, and Rajas on the table with the other ingredients for people to serve themselves family-style, or make each taco by putting about 2 ounces of the meat and Rajas in the tortillas and topping them with a little Guacamole and salsa.

Spicy Chicken Flour Tacos

4 servings, 2 tacos each

PER SERVING | 300 calories
17 g protein | 39 g carbohydrates
8 g total fat (3 g saturated)
35 mg cholesterol | 4 g fiber
2 g sugar | 230 mg sodium

I would put these simple, delicious tacos on any menu!

INGREDIENTS

1 pound Plain or Spicy Shredded Chicken or Turkey Filling (pages 122–123)
8 flour tortillas
4 ounces *queso fresco*, grated

DIRECTIONS

Heat the filling and reserve. Heat the tortillas in a large skillet or on a griddle over medium heat until they are hot and flexible. Fill each tortilla with 2 ounces filling, then top with the cheese.

Tacos al Pastor

SHEPHERD'S TACOS

4 servings, 2 tacos each

PER SERVING | 330 calories
23 g protein | 38 g carbohydrates
11 g total fat (1.5 g saturated)
65 mg cholesterol | 7 g fiber
9 g sugar | 610 mg sodium

These are the captivating tacos usually served as street food in Mexico from stalls, where the marinated meat is cooked on vertical skewers.

INGREDIENTS

4 slices canned pineapple, rinsed and dried
Extra-virgin olive oil, for the pineapple
8 hot corn tortillas
1 pound Shepherd's-style Pork Filling (page 114)
1 recipe Guacamole (page 59)
8 ounces Grilled Rajas (page 71), heated
Salsa

DIRECTIONS

Sear the pineapple in a pan filmed with a little oil over medium-high heat or sear in a grill pan. Chop the pineapple into small pieces and reserve.

Stuff the tortillas with the pork filling and top with a little Guacamole, some Rajas, some of the reserved pineapple, and salsa.

Tacos de Machacado

4 servings, 2 tacos each

PER SERVING | 450 calories | 25 g
protein
26 g carbohydrates | 26 g total fat
(8 g saturated) | 395 mg cholesterol
2 g fiber | 1 g sugar | 440 mg sodium

In Spanish, machacado *means "ground" or "crushed," and that is exactly how the dried beef called* carne seca *is processed before being made into what are perhaps the original and best breakfast tacos.*

INGREDIENTS

8 large eggs
6 ounces Carne Seca filling (page 116), about 1 cup loosely packed
3 tablespoons finely chopped cilantro
⅛ teaspoon salt
¼ teaspoon pepper
2½ tablespoons butter substitute
8 hot flour tortillas
¼ cup grated *cotija* cheese
Salsa

DIRECTIONS

Make the scrambled egg filling. Beat the eggs in a bowl just until the yolks and whites are combined. Stir in the Carne Seca, cilantro, salt, and pepper. Heat a large nonstick skillet over just over medium heat. Add the butter substitute and let it melt. Add the egg mixture to the skillet and stir with a rubber spatula or wooden spoon in long, sweeping motions until the eggs are done as you like them.

Make the tacos. Divide the cooked eggs and Carne Seca evenly among the tortillas, sprinkle on some cheese and salsa, and serve.

ENCHILADAS

The word *enchilada* comes from *enchilar*, "to season with chile." Although broad, it's a pretty good description. Because much of the cooking in Mexico in days gone by was done on stovetops without ovens, enchiladas were (and are) often prepared by giving corn tortillas a quick bath in hot oil to make them resistant to becoming soggy, then dipped into a red or green chile sauce, wrapped around a filling, and garnished with cheese and maybe some *crema*. If cooks wanted the sauce cooked into the tortillas, they first dipped them in the sauce and then into hot oil before filling them. In either case, they were often served without additional heating.

Immigrants to the United States found most living accommodations equipped with ovens and learned to cover the prepared enchiladas with more sauce or gravy, adding more cheese and baking them until bubbly. The following recipes use both approaches and include recipes spanning the breadth of enchilada possibilities.

Enchiladas Verdes

GREEN CHILE ENCHILADAS

4 servings, 2 enchiladas each

PER SERVING | 250 calories | 14 g protein
32 g carbohydrates | 8 g total fat
(1.5 g saturated) | 30 mg cholesterol
5 g fiber | 7 g sugar | 230 mg sodium

The name of these enchiladas comes from the fact that their sauce is made with fresh green chiles. The most common way to make them is to roll corn tortillas around a filling of shredded chicken and top them with a sauce of tomatillos and serrano or jalapeño chiles. This recipe is for that version. You will also find a recipe for delicious New Mexico–style Green Chile Enchiladas (page 135) made with the state's incomparable chiles.

The sauce can be made without any oil at all, but if you do that, it is best to heat the enchiladas very quickly in a microwave rather than in the oven to keep them from drying out. If you find the taste of the tomatillos overly tart, add additional water or cooking liquid and continue simmering the sauce until it reaches the proper consistency. The sauce can be made several days in advance and refrigerated.

For a vegetarian option, fill the enchiladas with one of the vegetarian fillings or tofu.

INGREDIENTS

For the sauce

2 small to medium serrano chiles, stems removed

3 cups water

1 pound tomatillos, husked and rinsed

¼ cup coarsely chopped cilantro

¼ cup coarsely chopped white onion

1 tablespoon extra-virgin olive oil

¼ teaspoon salt, or to taste

For the enchiladas

8 corn tortillas

Cooking spray

1 cup Plain or Spicy Shredded Chicken Filling (pages 122–123)

2 ounces *queso fresco*

DIRECTIONS

Make the sauce. Place the chiles in a saucepan, add about 3 cups water, bring to a boil, cover, and simmer for 10 minutes. Add the tomatillos, cover, and simmer until the tomatillos are cooked through but not falling apart, about 5 minutes. Remove the tomatillos and chiles from the pan and reserve the cooking liquid. Cool the chiles and tomatillos, then cut the chiles into small pieces and place them in a blender. Add the tomatillos, cilantro, and onions and blend for 10–20 seconds, or until the sauce is nearly puréed but still has some texture.

Heat the oil in a saucepan over medium heat, add the contents of the blender and ½ cup of the reserved tomatillo cooking liquid, and simmer for 10–15 minutes, or until the sauce is thick enough to coat the back of a spoon. Add the salt, cook another minute, and remove the pan from the heat.

Make the enchiladas. Preheat the oven to 350°F. Soften the tortillas (page 129). Place about 2 tablespoons of the chicken filling (about ¾ of an ounce) just off center on each one and roll. Place all the tortillas in a baking dish or 2 on each of four oven-proof plates. Top the enchiladas with the sauce, sprinkle with the cheese, and bake for 10 minutes, or until the cheese has melted and the sauce is bubbling. Alternatively, the enchiladas may be heated in a microwave for about 45 seconds on high. Serve with Coleslaw (page 97), rice or beans, or small portions of all three.

Enchiladas Verdes Estilo Nuevo México

NEW MEXICO–STYLE GREEN CHILE ENCHILADAS

4 servings, 2 enchiladas each

PER SERVING | 280 calories
13 g protein | 32 g carbohydrates
11 g total fat (3 g saturated)
35 mg cholesterol | 5 g fiber
6 g sugar | 460 mg sodium

In spite of the fact that it is low in both calories and fat, this version of one of New Mexico's best dishes is as good as any I have ever had. It combines the recipes for New Mexico-style Green Enchilada Sauce and Carnitas. I often make double batches of each one. That allows me to have Carnitas on one night, enchiladas on another, and to use the remaining ingredients to make items like omelets and tacos.

New Mexico has its own unique chiles and green chile sauces, and the basic recipe for this one came originally from Katie Meeks, who founded La Posta restaurant in Mesilla, New Mexico. It has many other uses, including for Huevos Rancheros Verdes, an omelet filling, and, when mixed with cheese, as a vegetarian filling for tacos and nachos or a topping for Mexican Pizzas. And what a joy that it turns out to be naturally low in calories and made almost entirely of good-for-you vegetables.

It is most authentic if made with New Mexico's Hatch chiles, but if they are not available, poblano or Anaheim chiles and a small amount of habanero pepper make a reasonable substitute. For that option, remove the seeds and veins from ½–1 habanero chile, chop it into small pieces, and blend it with the 1½ cups water that goes into the sauce. For a milder version, leave out the habanero.

Unfortunately, I have never found any decent-tasting canned green chiles, so you will need to roast and peel the fresh Hatch, poblano, or Anaheim chiles (page 16). ▸▸

For the sauce

1 tablespoon extra-virgin olive oil

1 teaspoon all-purpose flour

2 cloves garlic, minced

1½ cups roasted, peeled, and chopped Hatch green chiles,
　　or poblano or Anaheim chiles and the water blended
　　with habanero chile as described above

1 cup chopped white onion

½ cup chopped tomato

½ teaspoon salt

1½ cups water, or water blended with habanero chile
　　as described above

For the enchiladas

8 corn tortillas

Cooking spray

1 cup minced Carnitas (page 179), or 6 ounces part skim milk
　　mozzarella, grated

1 ounce mild cheddar cheese, grated

DIRECTIONS

For the sauce. Mix 1 teaspoon of the olive oil with the flour in a microwave-safe dish and microwave on High for 40 seconds. Stir and cool for about 15 seconds, then microwave again for 30 seconds. Reserve the roux.

Heat a saucepan over medium heat. Add the olive oil and garlic and cook just until the garlic has softened, about 30 seconds; do not allow it to brown. Add the chiles, onion, tomato, salt, and water and simmer for 10–20 minutes, or until most, but not all, of the liquid has evaporated. Stir in the roux, lower the heat, and simmer until the sauce is bound together and no longer watery.

Make the enchiladas. Soften the tortillas (page 17). Put about 2 tablespoons of the chopped Carnitas or ¾ of an ounce of mozzarella in a line just off center on each tortilla and roll the tortilla around the filling. The enchiladas can be made to this point several hours before serving and refrigerated.

Put 2 enchiladas side by side on each of four plates. Divide the sauce equally over the enchiladas and top with the cheddar cheese. Microwave each plate, separately, for about 45 seconds on High. Alternatively, you may bake them in a 350°F oven for about 10 minutes.

Interior-style Enchiladas

4 servings, 2 enchiladas each

PER SERVING | 220 calories
10 g protein | 29 g carbohydrates
7 g total fat (3 g saturated)
20 mg cholesterol | 3 g fiber
2 g sugar | 220 mg sodium

In Mexico, instead of using a lot of broth and then thickening the sauce with a roux of flour and butter or oil, as is regularly done in Mexican American cooking, red chile enchilada sauces are often simply reduced until they thicken naturally. The tortillas are dipped in the sauce, either before or after being softened in hot oil, and then rolled. These enchiladas are often served without a final heating in an oven or microwave.

INGREDIENTS

8 corn tortillas
1 cup Chile Sauce (page 45)
Cooking spray
8 ounces *queso fresco*, **shredded, or part skim milk mozzarella**

DIRECTIONS

Flavor and soften the tortillas. Place the tortillas on a work surface, brush the tops with Chile Sauce, then spray with cooking spray. Turn the tortillas over and repeat. Wrap the tortillas in a towel or put them in a microwave-safe tortilla warmer and microwave for about 35 seconds, or until they are very soft.

Roll the enchiladas. Put about ¾ of an ounce of cheese in a line just off center on each tortilla and roll the tortillas around the filling. The enchiladas can be made to this point and refrigerated for several hours before serving.

Heat the enchiladas. Place 2 enchiladas side by side on each of four oven-safe plates or place them all in a baking dish. Spoon a little of the remaining sauce over the enchiladas and top them with the remaining cheese. Microwave each plate, separately, for about 45 seconds on High, or until the cheese has melted and the sauce is bubbling. Alternatively, you may bake them in a 350°F oven for about 10 minutes.

Tex-Mex-style Red Chile Enchiladas

4 servings, 2 enchiladas each filled with beef picadillo

PER SERVING | 330 calories
19 g protein | 34 g carbohydrates
14 g total fat (5 g saturated)
35 mg cholesterol | 5 g fiber
3 g sugar | 470 mg sodium

Tex-Mex enchiladas are famous for their beef gravy sauces, usually made with ancho chiles. Although the sauce can be made with chile powder instead of dried ancho chiles, you lose the thickening quality of the whole chiles, which requires adding more roux (flour cooked in butter or oil) to obtain the same volume of sauce. Getting the right amount of beef flavor in the sauce is critical. You can experiment, but I suggest you begin by using the combination of beef broth and chile soaking liquid suggested below. The enchiladas are usually filled with either cheese or Beef Picadillo, with the latter, which are used for the nutrition calculations, having the fewest calories.

INGREDIENTS

For the red chile sauce

2 large ancho chiles, toasted and rehydrated (pages 15–16), with at least 1¾ cups of the soaking water reserved
4 large cloves garlic, chopped
1 teaspoon dried leaf oregano
1 teaspoon ground cumin
1¾ cups of the reserved chile soaking water
1½ cups low-sodium beef broth
1½ tablespoons butter substitute
1 teaspoon extra-virgin olive oil
¼ pound ground 96% lean ground beef
1½ tablespoons all-purpose flour
2½ tablespoons tomato sauce
¼ heaping teaspoon salt, or to taste

For the enchiladas

8 corn tortillas
Cooking spray
6 ounces Beef Picadillo (page 115), or mild cheddar cheese
¼ cup finely chopped white onion (optional)
2 ounces mild cheddar cheese, grated, for garnish

DIRECTIONS

Make the sauce. Place the chiles in a blender, add the garlic, oregano, cumin, and the reserved soaking liquid and blend until thoroughly puréed, about 2 minutes. Add the beef broth and blend again to combine. If there are any bits of chile skin left, put the sauce through a food mill or strainer to remove them. Reserve the mixture.

In a large saucepan over medium or just slightly lower heat, add the butter substitute and olive oil. Add the ground beef and cook, breaking it up with a spoon, until it is just cooked through. Add the flour and continue cooking, stirring constantly, for 4–5 minutes, turning the heat down as necessary to keep the flour from scorching.

Remove the saucepan from the heat and whisk about ½ cup of the blended chile mixture into the flour-meat mixture. When it thickens and any lumps disappear, add another ½ cup of the chile mixture then repeat until the liquid combines easily with no lumps. Place the pan on the heat, slowly whisk in the remaining blended liquid, add the tomato sauce, and bring to a very low simmer. Cook, stirring occasionally, until the sauce coats the back of a spoon, 20–30 minutes.

Preheat your oven to 350°F.

Make the enchiladas. "Soften" the tortillas (page 17). After the tortillas have been softened, place about ¾ of an ounce of either the Picadillo or the cheese just off center of each one, sprinkle on some onion, if using, and roll the tortillas into cylinders. Place all the tortillas in a baking dish or on four oven-safe plates.

Heat and serve the enchiladas. Top the enchiladas with the sauce, sprinkle with the cheese garnish and a little more onion, if you wish, and bake for 10–12 minutes, or until they are hot and the sauce is bubbling. Alternatively, the enchiladas may be heated in a microwave. Serve with rice, Refried Beans (page 67), and Coleslaw (page 97) or sliced lettuce and tomato.

Enfrijoladas

BEAN ENCHILADAS

4 servings

PER SERVING | 330 calories
10 g protein | 50 g carbohydrates
11 g total fat (2 g saturated)
5 mg cholesterol | 10 g fiber
5 g sugar | 360 mg sodium

The word enfrijolada *is a combination of the Spanish words for "beans" and "enchiladas," and that pretty well describes them. The beans take the place of both the usual filling and the sauce. Once you have the beans, the Enfrijoladas are quick and easy to make, but be sure to leave the beans fairly runny. While I usually do not like to substitute yogurt for cream, in this instance, a good whole milk yogurt works very well.*

INGREDIENTS

2¼ cups Refried Pinto Beans (page 67)
12 corn tortillas
Cooking spray
½ cup grated *cotija* cheese
Salsa
¼ cup minced white onion
2 tablespoons good-quality, creamy whole milk yogurt

DIRECTIONS

Soften the tortillas and make the Enfrijoladas. Soften the tortillas (page 16). Spread about 1½ tablespoons of beans on each side of each tortilla, fold them in half, then in half again to form triangles. Place 3 of them on each of four plates. Top the folded tortillas with the rest of the beans and add salsa and onions to taste. Sprinkle with cheese and garnish with a drizzle of yogurt. Microwave each plate of Enfrijoladas on High for about 40 seconds, or until they are very hot.

New Mexico–style Red Chile Enchiladas

4 servings

PER SERVING | 390 calories
14 g protein | 32 g carbohydrates
21 g total fat (8 g saturated)
25 mg cholesterol | 3 g fiber
3 g sugar | 440 mg sodium

I can never decide whether I like these or the Tex-Mex version best. I hope you will try them both. In New Mexico, enchiladas are often stacked rather than rolled, and that is what is called for in this recipe. It is not difficult to find dried New Mexico chiles, but it is hard to find really good ones outside the state. A convenient way of solving that problem is to order a delicious chile powder (page 10). While you will need to use a little more roux than with whole chiles, the flavor boost is worth the few extra calories.

INGREDIENTS

For the sauce

4 large cloves garlic or 6 small ones, peeled and coarsely chopped
¼ cup high-quality chile powder from New Mexico chiles
1 teaspoon dried leaf oregano
5 cups water
4½ tablespoons butter substitute
¼ cup all-purpose flour
2 bay leaves
2 teaspoons rice vinegar
¾ teaspoon salt, or to taste

For the enchiladas

8 corn tortillas
Cooking spray
6 ounces part skim milk mozzarella, grated
Reserved New Mexico–style Red Chile Sauce

DIRECTIONS

For the sauce. Place the garlic, chile powder, and oregano in a blender, add 1 cup of the water, and blend for 2 minutes. Add the remaining water and blend for 15 seconds. If your blender does not have a 5-cup capacity, just add however much it will comfortably hold, then add the rest of the water to the pot later.

Make the roux. Heat a large saucepan over just below medium heat. Add the butter substitute and, when it has just melted, stir in the flour with a whisk. Continue whisking until the roux turns the color of a brown paper bag, about 5 minutes. Remove the pan from the heat.

Add the broth. Pulse the broth ingredients in the blender to make sure they are still well mixed, then whisk about ½ cup of the broth into the roux. As soon as it is incorporated with no lumps, add another ½ cup. Repeat the process once or twice more, or until the liquid you are adding requires very little whisking. Return the pan to the heat and whisk in the remainder of the broth and any water that did not fit in the blender.

Finish the sauce. Bring the ingredients to a boil, lower the heat to a medium-low simmer, add the bay leaves and vinegar, and simmer until the sauce reaches the consistency of a thin-to-medium milkshake, 15–25 minutes. It should just coat the back of a spoon. Add salt to taste and cook another minute.

Assemble the enchiladas. Preheat your oven to 350°F. Soften the tortillas (page 17). Lay four of them flat on four oven-safe plates or on a large baking sheet. Sprinkle ¾ of an ounce of the cheese over each tortilla and top with the remaining tortillas. Top the enchiladas with the sauce, sprinkle with the remaining cheese, and bake for 10–12 minutes, or until they are hot and the sauce is bubbling. Alternatively, the enchiladas may be heated in a microwave. Serve with Pozole Side Dish (page 76) and a scoop of Frijoles de Olla (page 65).

Sweet Potato Enchiladas

4 servings, 2 enchiladas each

PER SERVING | 450 calories | 5 g protein
84 g carbohydrates | 11 g total fat
(2.5 g saturated) | 0 mg cholesterol
5 g fiber | 39 g sugar | 520 mg sodium

El Mirador restaurant in San Antonio, Texas, serves a delicious potato enchilada dish at dinner. Corn tortillas are filled with mashed potatoes, topped with a citrus reduction, and garnished with a salad mixed with mandarin oranges. After trying it, most people are hooked and often order nothing else. I had made a similar sauce and planned to include it in this book when I decided to try it with the Mashed Sweet Potato recipe (page 74). I think it turned out even better than the original and makes a knockout vegetarian meal. Nevertheless, feel free to substitute regular mashed potatoes. Reducing the sauce takes a little time but is well worth it.

This spectacular recipe is particularly good for entertaining or for family weeknight dinners. Do the potatoes, sauce, and dressing a day or two in advance, then all you have to do is roll the enchiladas, top them with a little sauce, heat them in a microwave, and garnish them with the salad, oranges, and cheese.

INGREDIENTS

For the citrus sauce
1 tablespoon extra-virgin olive oil
4 cloves garlic, peeled and minced, or put through a garlic press
2 cups apple juice
½ cup orange juice
½ cup pineapple juice
1 teaspoon chopped canned chipotle chile
2 teaspoons cider vinegar
2 teaspoons grenadine syrup
2 teaspoons agave nectar
¼ teaspoon dried thyme ▸▸

1 tablespoon cider vinegar

1 teaspoon Dijon mustard

2 teaspoons agave nectar

Pinch salt

Black pepper, to taste

1 tablespoon extra-virgin olive oil

For the enchiladas

8 corn tortillas, softened (page 17)

1½ cups Sweet Potatoes Mashed with Coconut Milk and Garlic
   (page 74)

Reserved citrus sauce

3 ounces lettuce or salad mix, chopped

Reserved salad dressing

1 cup mandarin oranges, drained, rinsed, and dried

2 tablespoons grated *cotija* cheese

DIRECTIONS

Make the citrus sauce. Heat the oil in a saucepan over medium heat and add the garlic. Just before it browns, add the remaining ingredients. Raise the heat to medium-high, bring the mixture to a boil, lower the heat to a simmer, and cook until the sauce just begins to thicken. At this point there should be about ½ cup remaining. Reduce the heat and continue cooking at a low simmer, stirring frequently, until the sauce is the consistency of a thin syrup. There should be about ⅓ cup. It is very easy to burn the sauce during the last few minutes, so be extra careful. Pour the reduction into a small dish and reserve. If the sauce becomes too thick, simply add a little more apple juice and heat in a microwave.

Make the salad dressing. Whisk all the ingredients except the oil in a small bowl. Whisk in the olive oil in a thin stream and reserve.

Assemble the enchiladas. Spread each tortilla with 3 tablespoons mashed sweet potatoes, roll, and put 2 of them on each of four microwave-safe plates. Spread about 1 tablespoon of the citrus sauce over each pair of enchiladas and microwave on High for about 35 seconds.

Toss the lettuce or salad mix with the dressing and mound it on top of the enchiladas. Divide the mandarin oranges equally among the plates and garnish with the cheese.

Enchiladas Sonorenses

SONORA-STYLE ENCHILADAS

4 servings

PER SERVING | 380 calories
12 g protein | 42 g carbohydrates
18 g total fat (10 g saturated)
20 mg cholesterol | 4 g fiber
2 g sugar | 929 mg sodium

Sonora-style enchiladas consist of very thick corn tortillas, almost like large gorditas, often with some cheese in the masa. They are covered with sauce and garnished with cheese, olives, and green onions. It is a shame this delicious rustic offering is not often found outside of Sonora, with the notable exception of Tucson's terrific El Charro restaurant. I used their recipe as a basis for this one, but changed it in several ways that I believe make the preparation easier but just as good. The enchiladas are authentic when made with lard, but the other choices also work well. It is difficult to give precise measurements for how much liquid to add to the dough because humidity plays a part. The masa needs to be just wet enough to come together and make smooth dough, but too much water will make the results soggy. Please note that the dish has more sodium than similar recipes, partially because of the baking soda, which has more salt than most people realize.

INGREDIENTS

For the masa

1⅓ cups Maseca corn flour for making corn tortillas
3 tablespoons potato flour
½ teaspoon baking soda
¼ heaping teaspoon salt
1½ ounces mild cheddar cheese, finely shredded
1 cup water
2 tablespoons lard, coconut oil, duck fat, or extra-virgin olive oil

To finish the enchiladas

2 cups shredded iceberg lettuce
1½ teaspoons rice vinegar
½ teaspoon dried leaf oregano
½ cup sliced black California olives
2 green onions, finely chopped
2 cups Chile Sauce made with New Mexico chiles (page 45)
2 ounces part skim milk mozzarella, grated

DIRECTIONS

Make the masa. In a bowl, mix the corn flour, potato flour, baking soda, salt, and cheddar cheese together. Stir in the water to form a dough. Knead for 2 minutes, cover the bowl with plastic wrap, and allow the masa to rehydrate for 30 minutes. Knead again until it is very smooth.

Form the dough cakes. Divide the dough into 4 balls of about 4 ounces each. Place one of them on a piece of plastic wrap and cover it with another piece of plastic. Using the bottom of a plate or a small skillet, press the dough into a ¼-inch-thick circle. Repeat with the remaining balls. ▸▸

Cook the masa. Preheat your oven to 150°F to keep the cooked masa warm unless you have a very large skillet or griddle that will accommodate them all. Heat a large skillet over medium heat, add half of the fat, and, as it melts, spread it over the entire surface of the pan. Peel the plastic wrap off 2 of the masa cakes and lay them in the skillet. Cook until the masa is golden brown on both sides and cooked through, about 6 minutes on each side. Repeat with the remaining masa. Keep the cakes warm in the oven until ready to assemble the enchiladas.

Finish the enchiladas. Combine the lettuce, vinegar, oregano, olives, and green onion and reserve. Place 1 masa cake on each of four plates. Heat the Chile Sauce to a boil and ladle some over each cake. Immediately sprinkle cheese over the hot sauce. Garnish the enchiladas with the reserved lettuce mixture.

Quesadillas de Elotes Asados y Rajas

ROASTED CORN AND RAJAS QUESADILLAS

4 servings, 1 quesadilla each

PER SERVING | 430 calories | 21 g protein 46 g carbohydrates | 19 g total fat (10 g saturated) | 35 mg cholesterol 5 g fiber | 7 g sugar | 800 mg sodium

QUESADILLAS

Quesadillas are corn or flour tortillas folded over cheese and other ingredients and cooked until the cheese melts. They can also be made flat, with the filling sandwiched between 2 tortillas. For appetizers or cocktail parties, cut quesadillas into small portions and serve on platters or trays.

The quantities in the following recipe are designed for the folded version. The dish can be made with frozen corn, but it will have a mushier texture. Both the corn and the Rajas can be prepared a day or so in advance and reheated in a microwave oven just before the final preparation. For the cheese, I suggest part skim milk mozzarella.

INGREDIENTS

2 ears of corn
¼ teaspoon salt
¼ teaspoon pepper
½ recipe Caramelized Rajas (page 70)
4 large, thin flour tortillas, about 8 inches in diameter
¼ cup sour cream
8 ounces part skim milk mozzarella
Salsa
Cooking spray

DIRECTIONS

Roast the corn. Husk the corn, remove the silk, and slice the kernels into a bowl. Heat a skillet (iron is perfect) over medium-high heat until it is very hot. Put the corn in the dry skillet and cook, stirring almost constantly, until the corn has patches of brown and begins to soften. This will take just a few minutes. Add the salt and pepper and mix the corn with the Rajas.

Make the quesadillas. On a large griddle or in a skillet over medium to medium-low heat, warm the tortillas. Place them on a flat surface next to the stove and brush the top of each with about 1 tablespoon sour cream. Keep the skillet warm as you assemble the quesadillas. Sprinkle about 1 ounce cheese over half of each tortilla and cover with some of the corn-Raja mix. Add another ounce of cheese, drizzle on some salsa, and fold the tortilla to cover the filling.

Spray the heated skillet or griddle liberally with cooking spray and cook the quesadillas until the bottom layer of cheese has melted and the bottoms of the tortillas are golden brown. Turn them over and repeat on the other side. Serve the Quesadillas with Guacamole (page 59) and additional salsa.

Mushroom Quesadillas

4 servings, 2 quesadillas each

PER SERVING | 410 calories | 21 g protein 34 g carbohydrates | 23 g total fat (10 g saturated) | 35 mg cholesterol 5 g fiber | 6 g sugar | 740 mg sodium

Combining the Mushroom Filling with Rajas, especially the caramelized version, makes for an exceptional quesadilla. Using two skillets will speed the preparation, but if you have only one, make the quesadillas in batches.

INGREDIENTS

8 (5- to 6-inch) corn or flour tortillas
¼ cup sour cream
8 ounces part skim milk mozzarella, grated, divided
⅔ recipe Mushroom Filling (page 120), heated
4 ounces Caramelized Rajas (page 70), heated
Salsa
Cooking spray

DIRECTIONS

Heat the tortillas. Heat one or two skillets or a large griddle over medium heat and warm the tortillas until they are heated through and very flexible. Keep the tortillas warm while you work. When you are finished, keep the skillets or griddle hot.

Lay the warm tortillas on a work surface and spread a little sour cream on each one. Spread ½ ounce cheese on half of each tortilla and top each with an equal amount of the Mushroom Filling, Rajas, and salsa. Sprinkle the remaining cheese over the Rajas and fold the tortillas firmly in half so they will stay folded.

Cook the quesadillas. Spray the hot skillets or griddle liberally with cooking spray and transfer the quesadillas to the pan(s). Cook the quesadillas over medium heat until the cheese has melted and the bottoms are turning golden, then turn them and cook until golden on the other side.

Spinach Quesadillas

4 servings, 2 quesadillas each

PER SERVING | 360 calories
16 g protein | 33 g carbohydrates
19 g total fat (7 g saturated)
30 mg cholesterol | 7 g fiber
4 g sugar | 710 mg sodium

This recipe is exceptionally easy once you have made the filling because it already contains cheese. I often serve the quesadillas cut into small pieces for appetizers. Using two skillets will speed the preparation, but if you have only one, make the quesadillas in batches.

INGREDIENTS

8 (5- to 6-inch) corn or flour tortillas
¾ recipe Spinach Filling (page 121)
Cooking spray

DIRECTIONS

Heat one or two skillets or a large griddle over medium heat and warm the tortillas until they are heated through and very flexible. Keep the tortillas warm while you work. When you are finished, keep the skillets or griddle hot.

Lay the hot tortillas on a work surface and top half of each one with an equal amount of the filling. Fold the tortillas firmly in half so they will stay folded.

Spray the hot skillets or griddle liberally with cooking spray and transfer the quesadillas to the pan(s). Cook the quesadillas over medium heat until the cheese has melted and the bottoms are turning golden, then turn them and cook until golden on the other side.

Huitlacoche and Mushroom Quesadillas

4 servings, 2 quesadillas each

PER SERVING | 350 calories
12 g protein | 33 g carbohydrates
19 g total fat (5 g saturated)
20 mg cholesterol | 5 g fiber
6 g sugar | 510 mg sodium

This recipe gets raves from Mexican food aficionados and could not be easier to prepare once you have the filling made.

INGREDIENTS

8 corn tortillas
Cooking spray
1 recipe Huitlacoche and Mushroom Filling (page 124)

DIRECTIONS

Heat one or two skillets or a large griddle over medium heat, then warm the tortillas until they are heated through and very flexible. Keep the tortillas warm while you work. When you are finished, keep the skillets or griddle hot.

Lay the hot tortillas on a work surface and top half of each one with an equal amount of the filling. Fold the tortillas firmly in half so they will stay folded.

Spray the hot skillets or griddle liberally with cooking spray and transfer the quesadillas to the pan(s). Cook the quesadillas over medium heat until the cheese has melted and the bottoms are turning golden, then turn them and cook until golden on the other side.

TOSTADAS

Tostadas are one of the easiest *antojitos* to prepare because once you have the shells and filling made, the rest of the preparation is minimal. You can make tostada shells by spraying a corn tortilla with a little cooking spray and baking it at 325°F for 15–20 minutes, or until crisp. It is a bit difficult to get them really crisp without overbrowning them, but after they come out of the oven, leave them to harden for about 15 minutes. If that does not work, try lowering the oven temperature to 300°F and cooking them a little longer. To me this method produces a tostada that doesn't have quite the correct taste and texture; however, some people do seem to like them, and the savings of about 80 calories per tostada is substantial. On the other hand, probably because of their fat content, flour tortillas are easier to bake and taste better. Spray them and bake at 350°F for about 8–10 minutes, depending on their thickness.

To make the tastier but fattier tostada shells with either corn or flour tortillas, simply heat about ½ inch canola oil in a small skillet to 350°F and fry the tortillas on both sides until they are crisp and then drain them on paper towels. For an incredibly crispy-crunchy treat, but one with more calories, make your tostadas by frying formed but uncooked flour tortilla dough.

Just about any of the fillings work well with tostadas, but I think my favorite is the Chorizo, Potato, and Carrots Filling. Beans, scrambled eggs, and cheese make a wonderful breakfast tostada. The following recipe is meant purely as a guide from which you can exercise your own imagination.

Basic Tostadas

4 servings, 2 tostadas each

PER SERVING | 190 calories | 6 g protein 20 g carbohydrates | 6 g total fat (1 g saturated) | 5 mg cholesterol 5 g fiber | 4 g sugar | 190 mg sodium

INGREDIENTS

8 corn tortilla tostada shells, prepared using one of the methods described above
½ cup Refried Beans (page 67)
¾ cup Chorizo, Potato, and Carrots Filling (page 120)
1 cup shredded lettuce
¾ cup chopped tomatoes
2 tablespoons shredded *cotija* cheese
Salsa

DIRECTIONS

Place 2 tostada shells on each of four plates and spread about 2 tablespoons of the beans on each one. Top with equal amounts of the Chorizo, Potato, and Carrots Filling, the lettuce, tomatoes, and cheese and serve with the salsa.

Gorditas de Papas

POTATO GORDITAS

About 16 gorditas. Nutrition information is for 1 gordita topped with a dab of guacamole. Calculations based on lard.

PER SERVING | 70 calories | 2 g protein
11 g carbohydrates | 2.5 g total fat
(0.5 g saturated) | 0 mg cholesterol
1 g fiber | 0 g sugar | 100 mg sodium

GORDITAS

The word *gorditas* means "little fat ones," and like so many other Mexican culinary terms, it is an accurate description. Gorditas are really small, fat corn tortillas that are often fried in lard.

I found the following gordita years ago in Nuevo Laredo's El Rincón del Viejo (The Old Man's Corner) restaurant. They quickly became my favorite gorditas and can serve as an appetizer or a light meal. The masa portion of the dough can be made either with fresh dough for corn tortillas from a tortilla factory or with Maseca corn flour for tortillas. It helps if you have a good food scale to correctly size the gorditas. A laser thermometer is also useful to make sure your griddle is at the proper temperature. Gorditas are traditionally cooked in lard, sometimes quite a bit of it. However, these use very little, so please consider using a good pure lard (page 12) for that special flavor.

INGREDIENTS

14 ounces prepared masa for corn tortillas, or 1½ cups Maseca and 1 cup plus 1 tablespoon water
9 ounces peeled russet potatoes (weighed after peeling), cut into 1½-inch chunks
2 teaspoons melted pure lard or butter substitute, plus a little more lard or cooking spray for frying the Gorditas
½ teaspoon salt
Pico de Gallo (page 46), or your favorite salsa
½ cup Guacamole (page 59)

DIRECTIONS

Prepare the masa. If you are using Maseca for tortillas, put 1½ cups in a medium-sized bowl and stir in 1 cup plus 1 tablespoon water with a wooden spoon. Knead the dough for about 2 minutes, or until it is quite smooth, then allow it to rest for 30 minutes, covered with plastic wrap, so that it will fully hydrate. The dough should weigh about 14 ounces.

Cook the potatoes and finish the dough. Place the potatoes in a pot, cover them with several inches of water, and simmer until they are easily pierced with a paring knife. Drain the potatoes and put them through a potato ricer or thoroughly mash them. Stir in the lard or butter substitute and salt. To finish the dough, combine the 14 ounces of tortilla masa and the mashed potato mixture.

Form the gorditas. Pat 1½-ounce pieces of the dough into circles. They should be between ⅛- and ¼-inch thick. Heat a nonstick skillet over medium heat (about 350°–375°F if you have a laser thermometer). Add just enough lard or cooking spray to film the surface and cook the dough until it begins to turn golden brown on the bottom, about 4 minutes. Turn the gorditas and cook another 4 minutes on the other side. Top them with a little Pico de Gallo, Guacamole, or just about anything else you like, and serve.

I am continually amazed at how re-gional Mexican food still is. Items that are extremely popular in some areas, such as puffy tacos in Texas and sopaipillas and flat enchiladas in New Mexico, remain difficult to find outside those areas. The Cheese Crisps and Mexican Pizzas found mostly in Ari-zona are yet another example. Usu-ally served as appetizers, light meals, or cocktail party fare, they are exactly what their names imply. They are best made with the paper-thin Sonora-style flour tortillas, which, if not avail-able in stores, can be made at home.

Cheese Crisps

4 servings as a light meal, 8 as an appetizer. Nutrition information is for 1 cheese crisp.

PER SERVING | 270 calories
16 g protein | 19 g carbohydrates
13 g total fat (6 g saturated)
30 mg cholesterol | 1 g fiber
0 g sugar | 590 mg sodium

Cheese Crisps are easy to whip up at the last minute, especially if you have properly thin flour tortillas. Several national brands produce them in 8-inch diameters. While making them from scratch takes more effort, they will be better and may have fewer calories.

INGREDIENTS

4 very thin 8-inch-diameter flour tortillas
8 ounces part skim milk mozzarella, grated
½ cup sliced, pickled jalapeño chiles

DIRECTIONS

Make the tortillas. If you decide to make your own tortillas, make the dough with the Basic Flour Tortilla recipe with the cake flour option (page 32) in order to make rolling out the tortillas as easy as possible. Use 1 cup of flour and divide and roll the dough into 6 equal balls of about 1.3 ounces each. Using a heavy rolling pin, roll the balls into 8-inch-diameter tortillas. Instead of cooking them on a very hot griddle, cook them over medium to low heat until they are just done on each side.

Preheat your oven to 375°F.

Bake the tortillas. Place the tortillas, whether purchased or homemade, directly on the oven racks and bake just until they become a bit stiff and begin to brown, 2–4 minutes.

Finish the cheese crisps. Remove the tortillas from the oven and top them with equal portions of the cheese and jalapeños. Return them to the oven until the cheese has melted, about 2–4 minutes. Remove the crisps from the oven with a large spatula and slice each one into 4 triangles.

Mexican Pizzas

These are basically Cheese Crisps with additional toppings, which, in addition to the cheese, can include just about anything that strikes your fancy. For a delightful vegetarian meal, try the following combination.

4 servings as a light meal, 8 as an appetizer. Nutrition information is for one pizza.

PER SERVING | 400 calories
19 g protein | 30 g carbohydrates
22 g total fat (10 g saturated)
35 mg cholesterol | 6 g fiber
4 g sugar | 580 mg sodium

INGREDIENTS

4 very thin 8-inch-diameter flour tortillas
8 ounces part skim milk mozzarella, grated
2 large poblano chiles, roasted, peeled, and chopped (page 16)
½ cup sliced black California olives
1 cup chopped tomatoes
1 large avocado, chopped
¼ cup sliced green onions, green part only
¼ cup loosely packed chopped cilantro
2 tablespoons sour cream
Arizona-style Salsa (page 41), or another favorite

DIRECTIONS

Prepare the Cheese Crisp recipe through baking the tortillas. After removing the partially crisped tortillas from the oven, brush them lightly all over with the salsa. Top the tortillas with equal amounts of the cheese, poblano chiles, olives, and tomatoes. Bake until the cheese has melted, 3–4 minutes. Remove the pizzas with a large spatula and top with the avocado, green onion, cilantro, and a few dabs of sour cream. Cut each pizza into 4 triangles and serve with more Arizona-style Salsa on the side.

TAMALES

Tamales that can be filled with almost anything imaginable are one of Mexico's most ancient dishes. The pre-Hispanic ones had little or no fat and were a bit dry. After the Spanish arrived, lard was added, which converted them to something resembling the proverbial food of the gods. Unfortunately, the amount of fat, even if something like coconut oil is substituted for lard, usually goes beyond what would be considered ideal. Except in one delightful case! When I lived in Arizona, I fell in love with what they call green corn tamales—tamales made not with masa from dried corn but with fresh corn and filled with mild green chile and cheese

Fresh Corn Tamales

About 12 tamales. Nutrition information is for 1 tamale.

PER SERVING | 120 calories | 5 g protein
15 g carbohydrates | 4.5 g total fat
(1.5 g saturated) | 20 mg cholesterol
1 g fiber | 5 g sugar | 230 mg sodium

The only difficulty in reproducing these mouthwateringly delicious tamales is that they are made not with sweet corn but with high-starch field corn. I tried various ways of mimicking the results obtained with field corn, such as adding dried corn masa to the fresh corn, but without much success. They were either too starchy or too runny—that is, until I adapted a recipe by Chef Mark Miller for Fresh Corn Tamales with Black Truffles and Black Truffle Butter. He used a combination of egg and cornmeal instead of starchy field corn to keep the tamales made with sweet corn from falling apart. When I replaced the truffles with green chile and cheese, the result was about as close to the delicious original as it needs to be.

Making tamales is much like baking, where ingredient amounts need to be precise, so I have given the measurements in both weight and volume. In addition to the ingredients below, you will need something in which to steam the tamales. You can buy tamaleras made for the purpose, or use bamboo steamers or something as simple as a fryer basket placed on something to raise it about 3 inches from the bottom of a large pot. The masa for these tamales is fairly runny, and rolling and tying them in traditional cornhusks requires some dexterity. But there is a nontraditional solution. Sealable plastic bags 6½ inches by 3¼ inches wide hold ¼ cup of the masa. Seal the bags and place them in the steamer. They don't look authentic, but they taste great!

INGREDIENTS

12 large dried cornhusks for making tamales, plus more to line
    the steamer basket

20 ounces of corn, or about 4 cups sliced from about 4–6 ears

½ cup cornmeal

½ teaspoon salt

1 teaspoon baking powder

¼ cup butter substitute, measured after melting

1 large egg plus one egg white from a large egg, beaten until light,
    about 30 seconds

1 tablespoon agave nectar

⅔ cup roasted, peeled, and minced poblano chiles (page 16)

3 ounces part skim milk mozzarella, grated

24 pieces of string cut into 5- to 6-inch lengths, or ¼-inch strips of
    cornhusks, or use good quality plastic bags that will not melt in
    the steamer, as mentioned above. ▸▸

Prepare the cornhusks. Put the cornhusks, if using them, in a pot, weight them down with something heavy, and cover them with hot tap water for at least 1 hour.

Make the masa. Put the corn in a blender and blend until it is puréed and smooth, about 1 minute. Pour it into a bowl and thoroughly mix in the remaining ingredients, except, of course, the string, cornhusk strips, or plastic bags.

Fill and tie the cornhusks. The masa is quite runny, so making the tamales is a bit awkward. First, place a layer of cornhusks in the bottom of your steamer basket. Wipe a rehydrated cornhusk dry with a towel and place it on your work surface. Pour ¼ cup of the masa down the center of the husk. Fold one long side over the masa, tuck the edge under the masa then roll the husk into a cylinder. Holding the rolled tamale in place with one hand, loop a piece of string or a cornhusk strip around the narrow end of the cylinder, about 1 inch up from the end, and, with the other hand, tie a knot to secure it. Tilt the tamale to allow the masa to run toward the knotted bottom and tie the top, just above the masa, probably an inch or 2 from the end. Place the tied tamale into the streamer basket. Fill and tie the remaining tamales in the same manner (or use the zipper bag solution mentioned above).

Steam the tamales. Place the steamer basket in a large pot on something that keeps it 3–4 inches from the bottom. Add enough water to come up to an inch or 2 below the steamer. Bring the water to a boil, cover the pot, and steam the tamales for 1 hour, keeping the water just below a boil. Put a penny in the pot to warn you by clanging if the water begins to evaporate. After an hour, turn off the heat and allow the tamales to continue steaming for 15 minutes.

Chiles Rellenos

4 servings

PER SERVING | 210 calories | 12 g protein
26 g carbohydrates | 7 g total fat
(1 g saturated) | 25 mg cholesterol
4 g fiber | 14 g sugar | 480 mg sodium

Like most antojitos, Chiles Rellenos can be filled with just about anything. One of my favorites is the Turks' Picadillo, and that is what the nutrition calculations are based on. However, the Minilla de Pescado, Carne Seca, Mushroom Filling, Spinach Filling, Plain or Spicy Shredded Chicken, or the Huitlacoche and Mushroom Filling are also good choices. I also like to add some roasted sweet potatoes with a little cheese.

Poblano chiles are most often used, but Anaheims are sometimes employed, as are dried anchos (see the recipe in Vegetarian Entrées, page 214). Most of us think of Chiles Rellenos as being deep-fried in an egg batter, or capeado, *as the process is called in Mexico. However, they are also made without the batter and just heated until soft and often served on a bed of rice. Besides being much lower in fat and calories, they are also much easier to make. In fact, for entertaining they can be made in advance, placed on a bed of rice, and heated in a microwave just before serving. What could be easier?*

INGREDIENTS

4 large poblano chiles, roasted, peeled, slit down one side, and
    seeded, stems left on (page 16)
2 cups filling of your choice
Cooking spray
1 cup Chile Sauce (page 45) or Yucatán-style Tomato Salsa
    (page 49), or salsa of your choice

DIRECTIONS

Preheat your oven to 375°F.

Stuff the peppers. Put about ½ cup filling in each pepper and spray the pepper with a little cooking spray. Place the stuffed peppers on a baking sheet and bake until they are soft; the exact time will depend on how soft they were after you roasted them. It can take anywhere from just a few minutes to 20 or more. Serve topped with the sauce or salsa.

POULTRY ENTRÉES

IN PRE-HISPANIC MEXICO, the only poultry available was wild game, such as duck, quail, and doves. The Spanish brought chickens and added another dimension to the developing cuisine.

Estofado de Pollo

A CHICKEN MOLE FROM OAXACA

I learned to make this outstanding dish at Oaxaca's Centro Cultural and, a few years ago, served it to raves at the San Antonio Heart Association formal gala event. Not your usual mole, *the recipe is a perfect example of a dish that is naturally healthful, although I do use Splenda as a substitute for sugar, and it works very well in that role. Of course sugar can be used in equal amounts.*

4 servings

PER SERVING | 400 calories
45 g protein | 26 g carbohydrates
16 g total fat (3 g saturated)
115 mg cholesterol | 6 g fiber
13 g sugar | 610 mg sodium

INGREDIENTS

1½ tablespoons extra-virgin olive oil

1¾ cups chopped white onions

4 cloves garlic, chopped

2 pounds tomatoes, very finely chopped (a food processor is a good choice for this)

4 ounces small to medium pitted green manzanilla olives (not stuffed with pimento), divided into 2 equal portions

2 ounces raisins, divided into 2 equal portions

2½ teaspoons Splenda

2¼ teaspoons dried thyme

Scant ½ tablespoon cinnamon, preferably *canela*

½ teaspoon salt

2 ounces blanched, slivered almonds, divided into 2 equal portions

4 canned pickled serrano chiles

1½ tablespoons pickled serrano juice from the can

2 tablespoons finely chopped parsley

4 (6-ounce) skinless, boneless chicken breasts

DIRECTIONS

Prepare the sauce. Heat 1 tablespoon of the olive oil over medium heat, add the onions, and cook, stirring often, until the onions are nearly soft. Add the garlic and continue to cook, stirring often, until it is cooked through but not browned, about 1 minute. Add the tomatoes and bring to a simmer. Add half of the olives and raisins and cook for 2 minutes. Add the Splenda, thyme, cinnamon, and salt and continue simmering for 5 minutes. Remove the pot from the heat and allow the contents to cool enough so they do not blow the top off the blender when you blend them. One way to prevent that is to remove the center piece of the blender's top and cover it with a towel, which allows steam to dissipate. In any case, be very careful, as severe burns can result from the steam and hot liquid.

    Blend, strain, and finish the sauce. Place the cooled ingredients and half of the almonds in a blender and purée. Strain the purée through the fine blade of a food mill or press through a strainer and pour it back into the pot. Bring it to a simmer and add the rest of the olives, raisins, and almonds. Add the chiles, chile juice, and parsley and simmer for 5 minutes. ▶▶

Cook the chicken and finish the recipe. Heat a nonstick sauté pan over medium-high heat, add the remaining ½ tablespoon of olive oil, then quickly brown the chicken on both sides. Add the sauce to the pan, stir, and simmer until the breasts are just cooked through. If the sauce becomes too thick, thin it with a little chicken broth or water.

I like it served over steamed squash with corn tortillas on the side or with rice.

Alambre de Pollo

NORTHERN MEXICAN
SHISH KEBAB

4 servings

PER SERVING | 260 calories
27 g protein | 8 g carbohydrates
13 g total fat (3 g saturated)
80 mg cholesterol | 2 g fiber
4 g sugar | 260 mg sodium

I found this delicious recipe in the northern Mexican village of Múzquiz in the state of Coahuila. It is really a splurge hidden in low-calorie clothing. The portions are ample, and it is good enough for entertaining. If you wish, you can leave out the small amount of bacon, but it adds a lot more flavor than fat to the dish. The result is most authentic and best when cooked over mesquite wood or charcoal on an outdoor grill. The sweet smoke turns it into something special. But it will also work well in a grill pan. If you choose the latter method, make sure your skewers are short enough to fit in the pan. This dish goes particularly well with Caesar Salad (page 96).

INGREDIENTS

For the marinade and chicken
⅓ cup freshly squeezed lime juice
1 tablespoon pure chile powder made from ancho or
　　New Mexico chiles
1 teaspoon salt
3 cloves garlic, minced
1½ teaspoons dried leaf oregano
¾ cup canola oil
1 pound boneless, skinless chicken breast, cut into 24 or 36 pieces

For the shish kebabs
1 large poblano chile, stemmed, seeded, and cut into ¾-inch pieces,
　　or substitute a bell pepper
1 white onion, cut into ¾-inch pieces
2 pieces bacon, cut into 24 pieces of about ¾ inch
4 small Roma tomatoes, cut into 3 pieces each
4 shish kebab skewers

Make the marinade and marinate the chicken. Combine the lime juice, chile powder, salt, garlic, and oregano, then slowly whisk or stir in the oil until well combined. Pour the marinade over the chicken in a nonreactive bowl and marinate for 1–1½ hours, but no longer, or the lime juice will begin to "cook" the chicken.

Parboil the chiles and onions. So that the chile and onion pieces will not be only partially cooked when the chicken is done, parboil them by immersing them in boiling water for about 5 seconds. Remove and rinse them under cold running water to stop the cooking. Drain and reserve.

Prepare the skewers. If using wood skewers, soak them in water for at least a half hour to keep them from burning. Thread the ingredients on the skewers in the following order (or any order you prefer): 1 piece pepper, 2 pieces onion, 1 piece tomato, 1 piece pepper, 2 pieces onion, 1 piece bacon, 2–3 pieces chicken (depending on how many you cut), 1 piece bacon, 2 pieces onion, etc.

Grill the shish kebabs. Prepare a wood or charcoal fire, start a gas grill, or put a grill pan on the stove to heat over medium-high heat. Grill the shish kebabs, turning them as each side browns, until the chicken is just cooked through.

Serve with Mexican Rice (page 61), Saffron Rice (page 62), or a Caesar Salad (page 96).

Pipián Verde

GREEN CHILE
CHICKEN STEW

4 servings

PER SERVING | 420 calories
47 g protein | 16 g carbohydrates
21 g total fat (4 g saturated)
115 mg cholesterol | 4 g fiber
7 g sugar | 430 mg sodium

Pipianes are a perfect example of how foreign ingredients—in this case, chicken, sesame seeds, cinnamon, orange juice, and oil—were absorbed into pre-Hispanic dishes. These simple stews, thickened entirely with their own ingredients rather than flour or cornstarch, are similar to the more complex moles. Both rely for their depth of flavor on cooking the ingredients separately and then combining them. Although this dish has a fair number of ingredients and steps, the process is simple—and well worth it for its intriguingly exotic taste.

Although pipianes are usually eaten as stews with corn tortillas, they are extremely versatile. Mixed with a few handfuls of crispy tortilla chips and topped with a little grated cheese, they become a terrific version of chilaquiles. They can also be made into enchiladas or used as fillings for tacos and burritos, or as a topping for tostadas. Please note that usually, but not always, 1 jalapeño makes the dish reasonably mild, 2 will be delightfully piquant, and 3 will be quite hot. ▸▸

¼ cup blanched, slivered almonds

¼ cup raw *pepitas* (page 13)

2 tablespoons sesame seeds

½ teaspoon whole cumin seeds

8 ounces tomatillos, cut in half

2 cloves garlic, unpeeled

1–3 jalapeño chiles

½ cup chopped white onion

1 corn tortilla

¼ teaspoon ground black pepper

1 teaspoon dried leaf oregano

½ teaspoon salt

¼ heaping teaspoon cinnamon, preferably *canela*

½ cup orange juice

1 tablespoon freshly squeezed lime juice

3 tablespoons extra-virgin olive oil

1¼ pounds boneless, skinless chicken breast, cut into ¾-inch pieces

1 cup low-sodium chicken broth

DIRECTIONS

Toast the ingredients. Toast the almonds in a skillet over medium heat until they begin to brown. Place them in a blender. Toast the pumpkin seeds in the same skillet until they pop like popcorn and add them to the blender. Toast the sesame seeds and cumin seeds in the skillet until the seeds turn golden and add them to the blender.

Raise the heat to medium-high and place the tomatillos in the pan cut side down. Add the garlic, jalapeños, and onions. After 3½–4 minutes, the bottoms of the tomatillos should be charred. Turn them and stir the garlic, jalapeños, and onions. Cook another 3½–4 minutes, or until everything is soft and charred. You may have to remove the onions early and leave the jalapeños in a little longer than the tomatillos. Remove the garlic, allow it to cool, then peel it and add it to the blender jar. Remove the jalapeños, remove their stems and seeds, and add the chiles to the blender with the tomatillos and onions.

Brush a little olive oil on both sides of the tortilla and toast it in the skillet on both sides until it begins to turn golden. Cut it into small pieces and add it to the blender.

Add the pepper, oregano, salt, cinnamon, orange juice, and lime juice to the blender and blend to a rough purée. The mixture should still have some body and texture.

Brown the chicken. Heat a Dutch oven or large pot over medium-high heat, add 1 tablespoon of the olive oil, and brown half of the chicken. With a slotted spoon, remove it to a bowl. Add another tablespoon of oil and brown the rest of the chicken. Return the first batch to the pot, lower the heat to medium, add the sauce, and cook, stirring constantly, for 1 minute. Stir in the broth, bring to a boil, lower the heat, cover the pot, and cook at a low simmer for 30 minutes. Remove the lid, raise the heat to produce a vigorous simmer, and continue to cook, stirring often, until the sauce has thickened.

Pollo Agridulce

SWEET-AND-SOUR CHICKEN

4 servings

PER SERVING | 400 calories
41 g protein | 12 g carbohydrates
22 g total fat (4 g saturated)
115 mg cholesterol | 3 g fiber
5 g sugar | 340 mg sodium

This is my version of a superb alta cocina *chicken dish I enjoyed at the Cien Años restaurant in Tijuana. If you like chile heat, you will love it! One caution: like all chiles, anchos come in differing degrees of heat. Although they are usually mild and slightly sweet, I once had some that brought tears. The only challenge is to finely chop the chiles. The older and harder they are, the more difficult it will be. Therefore, make sure you use very fresh, supple ones.*

INGREDIENTS

For the sauce
¼ **cup rice vinegar**
¼ **cup water**
¼ **heaping teaspoon salt**
5 **teaspoons sugar**
¼ **cup extra-virgin olive oil**
2 **cloves garlic, minced**
1 **cup (3–4) very fresh and supple ancho chiles, stemmed, seeded, and very finely chopped**

4 **(6-ounce) boneless, skinless chicken breasts pounded to about ½-inch thick**
½ **teaspoon kosher salt**
1 **tablespoon extra-virgin olive oil**

DIRECTIONS

Make the ancho chile sauce. Combine the vinegar, water, salt, and sugar in a cup and stir until dissolved. Heat a saucepan over medium to medium-low heat, add the olive oil, garlic, and chiles, and cook, stirring constantly, until the chiles begin to darken and stiffen, about 2 minutes. Add ½ cup of the vinegar mixture and simmer until about ⅔ of the liquid has evaporated. Set the sauce aside until you are ready to prepare the chicken. ►►

Cook the chicken. Season the chicken with the salt. Heat a nonstick skillet over medium-high heat, add the olive oil, and sauté the chicken until it is just done. If necessary, do this in batches to avoid crowding the chicken. Place the cooked chicken on serving plates.

Finish the sauce and serve. Bring the chile sauce back to a boil and simmer until it has thickened to a sauce-like consistency. Spoon the sauce over the chicken and serve with steamed vegetables.

Pozole Verde

POZOLE WITH GREEN CHILE

4 servings. Nutrition calculations were made with homemade hominy.

PER SERVING | 340 calories
32 g protein | 25 g carbohydrates
13 g total fat (3 g saturated)
70 mg cholesterol | 4 g fiber
6 g sugar | 300 mg sodium

Pozole is the Spanish word for hominy and refers to one of Mexico's most delicious but lesser known dishes. Somewhere in consistency between a soup and a stew, pozole is often named for the color of the chiles it is made with, usually red or green. It is served in bowls accompanied by various garnishes, the most unusual of which is crispy shredded iceberg lettuce. It makes an unexpectedly delicious addition, so be sure to try it. This terrific green chile version is easy to make and freezes well. If your chicken broth has a higher salt content than the one specified, simply reduce the amount of salt you add. It is best made with Homemade Hominy, especially if you are concerned with sodium. The dish can also be made with plain water or vegetable broth and with medium-hard tofu substituted for the turkey to make a vegetarian treat.

INGREDIENTS

1½ cups coarsely chopped tomatillos

2½ cups low-sodium (80 milligrams per cup) chicken broth

2 tablespoons extra-virgin olive oil

1 pound very lean ground turkey (3% fat)

1½ cups chopped white onion

2 cloves garlic, minced

¼ cup jalapeño chiles, cut into ¼-inch pieces

1 cup chopped green bell pepper

1½ cups cooked Homemade Hominy (page 11) or 1 (15½-ounce) can hominy, drained and rinsed

¼ heaping teaspoon salt

1 teaspoon dried leaf oregano

¼ teaspoon ground cumin

2 ounces *queso fresco*, shredded

1½ cups shredded iceberg lettuce

Lime wedges

Purée the tomatillos *with the broth*. Place the chopped tomatillos in a blender, add the broth and blend until completely puréed.

Brown the turkey. Heat a large pot or Dutch oven over medium-high heat, add 1 tablespoon olive oil, then add the ground turkey. Cook the turkey until it is just cooked through, stirring and chopping it constantly to break it into pieces as small as possible. Remove the browned turkey to a bowl.

Sauté the onion, garlic, and peppers. Turn the heat to medium, add the remaining 1 tablespoon oil, then add the onion, garlic, jalapeños, and bell pepper and cook, stirring frequently, until the vegetables are soft.

Complete the dish. Return the turkey to the pot. Stir in the hominy, the reserved tomatillo mixture, the salt, oregano, and cumin, and simmer, covered, for 30 minutes. Ladle the Pozole into bowls, sprinkle with cheese, and serve with lettuce and limes on the side.

Simple Mole

4 servings. Nutrition calculations are based on 6 ounces of skinless, boneless chicken breast per serving.

PER SERVING | 430 calories
46 g protein | 27 g carbohydrates
18 g total fat (3.5 g saturated)
115 mg cholesterol | 7 g fiber
11 g sugar | 460 mg sodium

When thinking of mole, *most people picture Puebla's* Mole Poblano, *the most famous of all. It is a superlative dish whose only disadvantage, besides requiring difficult-to-find mulato chiles, is that there are over 30 ingredients, and most of them require several stages of cooking. In an attempt to make that type of* mole *more accessible, Mexican restaurateurs and cookbook authors Alicia and Jorge De'Angeli published a recipe entitled* Mole Sencillo, Simple Mole. *After meeting them on a food tour of Puebla and Tlaxcala, I tried the recipe. It was indeed simple and also very good. While the following recipe is slightly more complicated, I think it is even better and still very easy to prepare.*

INGREDIENTS

3 ounces ancho chiles (5–6 medium to medium-large), weighed with
    seeds and stems, toasted, seeded, and rehydrated (pages 15–16)
½ tablespoon toasted sesame seeds
3 tablespoons blanched, slivered almonds
2 tablespoons raisins
1 cup chopped white onion
½ teaspoon cinnamon, preferably *canela*
½ teaspoon dried leaf oregano
3 cups low-sodium chicken broth, approximately
2½ tablespoons lard or olive oil, or a combination
1 teaspoon agave nectar
½ teaspoon salt, or to taste
2 tablespoons Mexican chocolate, finely chopped
1½ pounds cooked chicken, turkey, or pork ▸▸

Toast the sesame seeds and blend the sauce ingredients. While the chiles are soaking, toast the sesame seeds in a dry skillet over medium heat until they just turn golden brown. Place the rehydrated chiles in a blender. Add the sesame seeds and then add the almonds, raisins, onion, cinnamon, oregano, and ½ cup of the broth. Blend the ingredients for 2 minutes, adding a little more broth if necessary for the blender to operate. If the mixture is not totally smooth, put it through the fine blade of a food mill or a strainer.

Cook the sauce and finish the dish. Heat the lard or oil in a medium-sized pot over just above medium heat. Add the blended ingredients and cook, stirring constantly, until very thick and the paste becomes shiny as it releases its fat. Little by little, stir in the remaining broth and add the agave nectar. At this point the mixture should be thinner than you want the finished sauce to be. If necessary add some more broth. Simmer the sauce for about 15 minutes, until it is the consistency of a milk shake, add the salt and Mexican chocolate and serve over cooked chicken, turkey, or pork.

Grilled Chicken or Fajita-style Chicken

4 servings

PER SERVING | 230 calories
40 g protein | 7 g carbohydrates
5 g total fat (2 g saturated)
115 mg cholesterol | 2 g fiber
3 g sugar | 610 mg sodium

This recipe is about as easy as one this good can be, even if you decide to use the marinade and Rajas. If you plan to serve the chicken fajita-style—that is, sliced into bite-sized pieces—the breasts should be about ½-inch thick. If they are reasonably close to that, all you need to do is put them between two sheets of plastic wrap and gently pound them with a meat pounder or the bottom of a small, heavy iron skillet until they are the proper thickness and uniformly thick all over. If the breasts are very thick, as many are these days, you will need to slice them horizontally into two thinner pieces and then pound them a bit to even them out. If possible, I suggest you at least try the marinade, as it adds an extra dimension to what is normally a fairly bland ingredient.

INGREDIENTS

1½ pounds boneless, skinless chicken breast
Marinade from the recipe for Grilled Top Sirloin (optional, page 174)
½ teaspoon kosher salt
Black pepper, to taste
1 recipe Grilled Rajas (optional, page 71)

DIRECTIONS

If you are using the marinade, marinate the chicken for at least 3 hours in the refrigerator. Whether you are using the marinade or not, season the chicken with salt and pepper and grill it over hot coals or on a hot gas grill until it is just cooked through. If serving the chicken fajita-style, slice the meat crosswise into ½-inch pieces and toss it with the Rajas, if you're using them. Serve with hot tortillas, Guacamole (page 59), and salsa.

Pollo Pibil

YUCATÁN PIT-STYLE
CHICKEN

4 servings

PER SERVING | 220 calories
29 g protein | 15 g carbohydrates
6 g total fat (1.5 g saturated)
75 mg cholesterol | 4 g fiber
7 g sugar | 510 mg sodium

This traditional Yucatecan dish was originally prepared in earthen pits. These days it is usually baked in ovens, at least in most restaurants, and that is what this recipe calls for. However, you can easily make it using the indirect method in a covered charcoal grill and you will get that extra kiss of smoke, although the fire-roasted tomatoes and smoked paprika do add some smoke to the flavor. Traditionally, individual pieces of skin-on, bone-in chicken are rubbed with the seasoning paste, wrapped in banana leaves, and then cooked. I tried making the dish with cut-up skinless, boneless chicken breasts and was pleasantly surprised with the result, so that is what the recipe calls for.

Two shortcuts are available. You could use packaged achiote paste instead of making the rub yourself, and you could forget the banana leaves and just use foil. However, the taste will be less assertive and less interesting with commercial paste, and if you leave out the banana leaves, you will miss an entire taste dimension. While most recipes include plain paprika, I have specified hot smoked Spanish paprika for the extra heat and flavor, but feel free to substitute regular sweet paprika and to add a little cayenne for heat.

INGREDIENTS

For the rub
½ tablespoon annato seeds, ground to a powder in a spice or
   coffee grinder
1 teaspoon dried leaf oregano
¼ teaspoon ground cumin
½ teaspoon hot smoked Spanish paprika
¼ teaspoon cinnamon, preferably *canela*
¼ teaspoon ground allspice
½ teaspoon ground black pepper
¼ heaping teaspoon salt
4 cloves garlic, minced or put through a garlic press
1 tablespoon freshly squeezed lime juice
1 tablespoon orange juice

1 pound skinless, boneless chicken breasts, cut into 1-inch pieces
Reserved rub

For the sauce

1 tablespoon extra-virgin olive oil

1 cup chopped white onion

1 (14½-ounce) can diced fire-roasted tomatoes, liquid drained and
  discarded

⅛ teaspoon salt

1½ tablespoons chopped cilantro

2 strips of banana leaf, 8–12 inches wide by 2 feet long,
  softened (page 6)

Butcher twine

Aluminum foil

DIRECTIONS

Make the rub. Combine the dry ingredients, add the garlic, and stir in the juices to make a paste. Reserve.

Marinate the chicken. In a nonreactive bowl, massage the rub into the chicken by hand. I suggest wearing rubber gloves, as the annatto seeds can stain. Refrigerate the chicken for at least 3 hours or overnight.

Make the sauce. Preheat your oven to 350°F. Heat the oil in a saucepan over medium heat. Cook the onion until it just begins to soften, 3–4 minutes. Add the tomatoes and salt and simmer until the liquid is quite thick, 6–8 minutes. Stir in the cilantro and remove the saucepan from the heat. Allow the mixture to cool.

Wrap the chicken. Place the two softened banana leaves on a work surface, shiny side up, one across the other in the shape of a cross. Spread half the sauce in an 8-inch-diameter circle in the center of the cross. Mound the chicken over the sauce and top it with the remaining sauce. Fold the top leaf over the chicken as tightly as possible then do the same with the bottom leaf. Hold the package closed with one hand and slide a long piece of string under it with the other. Use the string to secure the package as you would wrap a gift, and then wrap the whole thing in a piece of aluminum foil. Place the package on a baking sheet in case it leaks. Bake 40 minutes. Remove the package to a serving platter, bring it to the table, and open it in front of the diners.

Grilled Quail

4 servings

PER SERVING | 260 calories
40 g protein | 0 g carbohydrates
10 g total fat (2.5 g saturated)
130 mg cholesterol | 0 g fiber
0 g sugar | 330 mg sodium

Grilled quail is popular in northern Mexican cooking, is easy to prepare, and makes a delicious, healthy meal. I particularly like it with the marinade used in the Grilled Top Sirloin recipe, but feel free to use your own—or none at all. For a knockout upscale meal, I serve the quail with the Cranberry-Jalapeño Jelly and the Quinoa. Nutrition calculations do not include the jelly or the quinoa. One tablespoon of the jelly would add about 35 calories, and a ½-cup serving of the quinoa, about 110 calories.

INGREDIENTS

8 quail, partially deboned, if possible
1 recipe of marinade for Grilled Top Sirloin (page 174)
½ teaspoon kosher salt
½ teaspoon ground black pepper
Cranberry-Jalapeño Jelly (optional, page 52)
Quinoa (optional, page 79)

DIRECTIONS

Marinate and grill the quail. Marinate the quail in a plastic zipper bag or a bowl, refrigerated, for at least 3 hours or overnight.

Prepare a charcoal or wood fire in the grill or heat a gas grill or a grill pan to high heat. Season the quail with the salt and pepper and grill it on both sides until just cooked through. Serve with a little of the jelly and the quinoa, if you wish.

Sinaloa Chicken

4 servings

PER SERVING | 280 calories
41 g protein | 7 g carbohydrates
10 g total fat (3 g saturated)
115 mg cholesterol | 1 g fiber
1 g sugar | 240 mg sodium

For some reason, the proprietors of food stalls in cities and roadside stands in the state of Sinaloa focus on preparing spicy grilled chicken, probably because it is incredibly popular. The dish usually consists of a whole butterflied chicken that is marinated and grilled. Often the marinade is a simple but spicy concoction of vinegar, orange juice, chile powder, and spices. But others, such as the one I tried on the outskirts of Mazatlán, are more complex—and interesting. Usually I rebel against recipes that are light versions of the original, and in this case the argument for the original is potentially strong. After all, isn't the crispy skin the main attraction of roasted or grilled chicken? That would normally be so, but in this case, the light version has so much of the taste of the original and definitely provides that all-important reward that makes me look forward to having it again and again that I have no problem giving crispy skin a pass. Cooking a large, skinless, boneless breast with the thick marinade over very hot coals gives the chicken a charred, crusty exterior, while the interior remains tender and juicy. No, it's not crispy golden-brown skin, but it's very good and has relatively few calories and not much fat.

INGREDIENTS

For the marinade

4 ounces tomatillos (2–3), cut in half
5 cloves garlic, unpeeled
2 (½-inch) slices of white onion, about 2 ounces
1 Anaheim chile, roasted and peeled (page 16)
1 teaspoon ground cumin
½ teaspoon salt
1 teaspoon cinnamon, preferably *canela*
½ teaspoon ground cloves
1 teaspoon ground allspice
1½ tablespoons pure ancho chile powder
1½ teaspoons piquín chiles
⅔ cup orange juice
2 tablespoons cider vinegar
2 tablespoons agave nectar
½ tablespoon lower-sodium soy sauce
¼ cup canola oil

Reserved marinade (with added canola oil)
1½ pounds large (about ½ pound each) boneless, skinless chicken breasts

For the sauce

2 tablespoons butter substitute
½ cup chopped white onions
Reserved ½ cup marinade (without added canola oil)
1 cup low-sodium chicken broth

DIRECTIONS

Make the marinade. Heat a skillet over medium to medium-high heat, add the tomatillos, cut side down, the garlic, and the onion slices and cook until the tomatillos are well charred on the bottom, 3½–4 minutes. Turn the tomatillos and stir the other ingredients and cook another 3½–4 minutes. Remove the garlic to a plate until cool enough to peel. Add the peeled garlic, tomatillos, and onions to a blender. Put the remaining marinade ingredients in the blender and purée. Reserve ½ cup of the marinade to make the sauce. Stir the canola oil into the remaining marinade.

Marinate the chicken. Marinate the chicken in a large zipper bag or nonreactive bowl, refrigerated, for at least 3 hours or overnight.

Make the sauce. Melt the butter substitute in a small saucepan over medium heat. Cook the onions, stirring frequently, until they are golden brown, adjusting the heat as necessary to keep them from scorching. Add the reserved ½ cup marinade and cook, stirring frequently, until it thickens. Stir in the chicken broth, raise the heat to medium-high, and continue cooking, stirring occasionally, until the sauce is thick enough to hold its shape.

Grill the chicken. Prepare a charcoal or wood fire or heat a gas grill or a grill pan as hot as possible and grill the chicken for about 2 minutes. Turn and continue grilling until the chicken is charred on the outside and no longer pink but still moist on the inside. Serve topped with a little of the sauce.

BEEF ENTRÉES

BEEF IS USED in all parts of Mexico but is the king of foods in northern Mexico, a heritage of the immense haciendas and the vaqueros of bygone days. For years, Mexico's grass-fed beef was maligned for lack of tenderness, but, recently, people have begun to understand that it is a healthier option than corn-fed beef. Fortunately, tender, high-quality grass-fed beef is now increasingly available in the United States.

Santa Maria–style Tri-tip Steak

6 servings

PER SERVING | 360 calories
36 g protein | 3 g carbohydrates
22 g total fat (7 g saturated)
115 mg cholesterol | 1 g fiber
0 g sugar | 570 mg sodium

Some of the earliest Mexican cooking in the United States began in California before Mexico's independence from Spain. The Californios of central and northern California created delicious Mexican-style foods, and it is a shame that more of them have not been revived. However, one specialty from the area that is in no danger of being ignored is the delicious and relatively low calorie cut of meat called a tri-tip. Although it is less tender than, say, a New York cut, it is the overwhelming choice of pit masters in the area around Santa Barbara and Santa Maria. There, the steak is seasoned with a special rub and seared on both sides over hot red oak coals. It is then smoked over lower heat until medium-rare. Around Santa Maria, they use barbecues whose grills can be raised and lowered in relation to the coals. They are terrific, but the dish can also be prepared on the more common kettle-style grill, and that is what this recipe describes. The tri-tip is similar to a top sirloin, which makes a decent substitute.

INGREDIENTS

7 tablespoons extra-virgin olive oil
4 cloves garlic, roughly chopped
1 tablespoon freshly ground black pepper
1 tablespoon granulated garlic
1 teaspoon granulated onion
½ tablespoon smoked or sweet Spanish paprika, or regular paprika
½ teaspoon smoked hot Spanish paprika, or cayenne
½ tablespoon kosher salt
½ tablespoon coarsely chopped fresh rosemary leaves
½ tablespoon dried parsley
2–2½ pounds tri-tip steak, or substitute top sirloin cut 2–2½ inches thick
¼ cup red wine vinegar

DIRECTIONS

Make the garlic-infused oil. Mix the olive oil and garlic in a microwave-safe dish and microwave on High for 45 seconds. Allow the garlic to infuse the oil for 1 hour, then strain out the garlic and reserve the oil. There should be about 6 tablespoons.

Make and apply the rub. Combine the black pepper, granulated garlic, granulated onion, both paprikas, salt, rosemary, and parsley. Brush both sides of the steak with 2 tablespoons of the garlic-infused oil. Sprinkle half the rub on one side of the meat and massage it in with your fingers. Repeat on the other side. Allow the steak to sit, refrigerated, for 3 hours or overnight before grilling.

Make the basting liquid. Mix ¼ cup of the garlic-infused oil with the red wine vinegar and reserve. ▶▶

Build the fire. Fill and light a charcoal starter with red oak, another kind of oak, or charcoal. If you do not have oak wood, if possible soak two handfuls of oak smoking chips for at least 20 minutes before grilling. In either case, when the coals are nearly ready, dump them into one side of your barbecue. Heat the grill for 5 minutes then clean it with a grill brush.

Grill the meat. Using kitchen tongs, run a paper towel soaked in vegetable oil over the grill and then put the steak (fat side up) directly over the hot coals. Grill the meat, uncovered, until it is a crusty dark brown on both sides, about 4 minutes per side. Move the meat to the side of the grill, away from the coals. If you are using charcoal, drain the soaked oak chips and place them on the coals. Brush the meat with the basting liquid, cover the grill, and smoke the meat, turning and basting it every 5 minutes until it is about 133°F for medium-rare. The entire process should take about 30 minutes. When the meat is done, remove it to a plate, tent it loosely with foil, and allow it to rest for 10 minutes. Slice the meat against the grain into ¼-inch slices. To keep the meal traditional, serve the steak with Santa Maria–style Beans (page 68).

Filete Sonorense

SONORA-STYLE
TENDERLOIN

4 servings

PER SERVING | 220 calories
33 g protein | 2 g carbohydrates
10 g total fat (2.5 g saturated)
90 mg cholesterol | 0 g fiber
0 g sugar | 780 mg sodium

I named this steak for the beef-raising state of Sonora, where I have most often found it and because that's what it was called in a Baja California restaurant I frequented. It consists of the whole center of the tenderloin grilled slowly over coals. I like to use mesquite wood, as it does not burn quite as hot as mesquite charcoal, but either works, as will ordinary briquettes with the addition of soaked mesquite chips. The tenderloin is the tenderest and one of the leanest beef cuts, and it is one of the only ones that combine those qualities. It is often criticized for a lack of beefy flavor, and in Mexico it is usually cooked with no more seasoning than salt, pepper, and a squeeze of lime juice. But in one Sonora restaurant the chef used a delicious paste that kicked up the flavor without seeming artificial. I often use the paste with choice tenderloin, but with prime meat I think the natural flavor, combined with the incomparable effect of the mesquite smoke, is sufficient.

INGREDIENTS

For the flavoring paste

¼ teaspoon salt

4 large cloves garlic, minced

1 tablespoon adobo sauce from a can of chipotle chiles

1 teaspoon low-sodium soy sauce

1 teaspoon freshly squeezed lime juice

For the steak

1½ pounds whole beef tenderloin, cut from the center

Reserved flavoring paste (optional)

2 tablespoons extra-virgin olive oil

1 teaspoon kosher salt

Ground black pepper, to taste

Mesquite wood, mesquite charcoal, or briquettes and
    soaked mesquite chips

DIRECTIONS

Make the flavoring paste. Place all the ingredients for the flavoring paste in a *molcajete* or mortar and pestle and grind to a paste.

Prepare the steak. If you are using the flavoring paste, brush it all over the steak about 3 hours before cooking and refrigerate. Whether you use the flavoring paste or not, about an hour before cooking, brush the entire steak with the olive oil and season with salt and pepper.

Grill the steak. If you are using mesquite chips, cover them with water 20 minutes before cooking. Allow the coals to burn to the point that they are not quite raging hot. The goal is to grill the steak fairly slowly for a total of 30–35 minutes for medium-rare, so check frequently. If the underside is quite charred after 2½ minutes, the coals are a little too hot, so move the meat to one side. Continue grilling, giving the meat a quarter turn at least every 5 minutes, until it is done as you like it. After grilling, allow the steak to sit for 10 minutes under a loose aluminum foil tent, then cut it into 4 pieces and serve.

Imperial Valley Carne Asada

4 servings

PER SERVING | 190 calories
24 g protein | 1 g carbohydrates
10 g total fat (3.5 g saturated)
75 mg cholesterol | 0 g fiber
0 g sugar | 970 mg sodium

Like many rural border areas, California's Imperial Valley has its own culture, and its unique Carne Asada is a great example. The recipe was originally made with flank steak, later with skirt steak, and recently with loin flap meat that is cut and pounded thin and marinated with lemony concoctions for at least 24 hours. Produced mostly by small independent grocery stores in El Centro, Brawley, and Heber, the recipes are carefully guarded secrets.

Unimpressed after trying Internet versions purporting to be the real thing, I went to the source. At each market I bought a steak and grilled it for dinner. Each was slightly different, but they all had an interesting balance of citrus and salt, and all of them were significantly better than the Internet recipes. After a lot of questions and a few tries, I was able to come very close to my favorite version, the one sold at Kennedy Market in Heber. The biggest problem was that I wanted to use flank steak because it is so lean. It is also tough and better suited to braising than grilling. Instead of using a commercial tenderizer, all of which include spices that give an unpleasant artificial taste, I turned to the more natural tenderizer often used in Chinese cooking: baking soda. That, an initial salting, and some pounding and manual tenderizing with a fork (or one of the spring-loaded devices with thin, razor-sharp blades) worked well. You could buy machine-tenderized flank steak, but it is more difficult to cut to the proper thickness and will have a poorer texture. I know that ¼ pound per person doesn't seem like much, but the steaks are so thin and so highly seasoned that they give the illusion of being much larger. Although it is high in sodium because of the baking soda and marinating, the recipe is so unusual and low in calories that I find it an interesting treat.

INGREDIENTS

1 (1-pound or a little more) flank steak, fairly thin
3 teaspoons salt
1½ teaspoons baking soda
¼ cup orange juice
½ cup fresh lemon juice
¼ cup water
¼ teaspoon black pepper
½ teaspoon dried leaf oregano
1 tablespoon dried cilantro
4 cloves garlic
½ medium-sized serrano chile, chopped
Zest of 2 lemons
2 tablespoons canola oil

DIRECTIONS

Slice and pound the meat. The steak will probably be somewhere between ½- and ¾-inch thick. The first task is to cut it into 2 pieces that will be between ¼- and ⅓-inch thick, and that is easier than you might think. It is particularly easy if the meat is partially frozen. Lay the meat on your work surface and hold the blade of a long, very sharp knife in the middle of one of the short ends of the meat, parallel to the work surface. Keeping the knife parallel, carefully slice the meat in half to form the two thinner pieces. You will need to hold the meat firmly in place with your other hand, so make sure you keep it even with, or behind the knife's cutting edge to avoid being cut if you make a mistake. Place each piece of meat on the work surface between two sheets of plastic wrap and pound to less than ¼ inch with a meat mallet or the bottom of a small iron skillet.

Salt and tenderize the meat. Using a total of 2 teaspoons salt, season both sides of each piece of meat and refrigerate it for 1½ hours. Rinse as much salt as possible from the meat and dry it with paper towels. Sprinkle an equal amount of the baking soda over both sides of each piece of meat and rub it in with your fingers. With a fork or, much better, with one of the tenderizing devices mentioned above, jab the meat repeatedly on each side. This will make the meat still thinner and tenderize it without ruining the texture. Place the meat in a glass bowl or large zipper bag.

Marinate the meat. Put the juices, water, pepper, oregano, cilantro, garlic, serrano, and remaining 1 teaspoon salt into a blender and purée. Stir in the lemon zest and oil. Pour the marinade over the meat in a zipper bag or nonreactive bowl (covered), and refrigerate for 24 hours.

Grill the meat. Remove the meat from the marinade, dry it thoroughly, and scrape off any of the dried cilantro. Heat the grill as hot as it will get, brush the meat with the oil, and grill it to medium-rare.

Grilled Top Sirloin

4 servings

PER SERVING | 200 calories
33 g protein | 0 g carbohydrates
8 g total fat (2 g saturated)
95 mg cholesterol | 0 g fiber
0 g sugar | 330 mg sodium

Top sirloin is a terrific choice in terms of taste, tenderness, calories, fat, and price. It is also easy to grill. However, this recipe is almost more about the marinade than the meat. Putting aside the debate advanced by some of my northern Mexican friends as to whether marinades should be used at all with beef, I have long searched for one that will do no more than enhance the natural flavor and do that well. While I previously published the marinades I liked at the time, I always had the feeling that something was missing—until this one, which has the added advantage of pairing well with chicken, pork, and even fish. It intentionally uses very little salt and no black pepper, so those can be applied as usual just prior to grilling. The end result is especially sensitive to changes in the amount of soy sauce (which enhances browning) and lime juice, so if you want a less bold result, just use a little less of them.

Marinated or not, the top sirloin is a great cut to make everything from a steak entrée to an al carbón (charbroiled) filling for tacos or burritos and is much leaner and a good substitute for the skirt steak used to make fajitas. It also heats up well in a microwave at half power. If you plan to do that, I suggest you leave it a little more rare than usual when you grill it.

INGREDIENTS

For the marinade
2 cloves garlic, chopped
½ tablespoon pure ancho chile powder
¼ teaspoon salt
1 tablespoon chopped canned chipotle chile
½ tablespoon lower-sodium soy sauce
½ teaspoon Worcestershire sauce
½ tablespoon freshly squeezed lime juice
½ cup canola oil

Reserved marinade, if using
1 very lean choice top sirloin steak fillet, 1¼ pounds,
    cut ¾- to 1-inch thick
½ teaspoon kosher salt
Black pepper, to taste

DIRECTIONS

Make the marinade (optional). Put all the marinade ingredients in a blender and purée, about 1 minute.

Marinate the steak (optional). Put the steak and marinade in a zipper bag and refrigerate for at least 3 and up to 24 hours.

Grill the steak. Season both sides of the steak with salt and pepper and grill it over a hot fire, turning it once, until it is as done as you like it.

Steak Tampiqueña

4 servings

- ▸ ½ cup Mexican Rice
  (page 61; 220 calories)

- ▸ ½ cup Refried Beans
  (page 67; 160 calories)

- ▸ 1 Spinach Quesadilla
  (page 146; 180 calories)

- ▸ 1 Interior-style Enchilada
  (page 137; 110 calories)

- ▸ ¼ recipe of one of the
  Rajas (pages 70–71;
  Grilled, 30 calories;
  Seared, 110; or
  Caramelized, 150)

- ▸ ¼ recipe Guacamole
  (page 59; 80 calories)

This popular dish was invented by famous restaurateur José Inéz Loredo. He moved from Tampico to Mexico City in 1929, where he opened the famous Tampico Club and served the steak he had learned to prepare in his hometown. Like so many things in the food world, there is controversy about the composition of the original dish. Whichever version is correct, Steak Tampiqueña has evolved into a glorious combination plate, where everything is optional except the specially cut thin steak, traditionally tenderloin, that is served with various antojitos, beans, rice, and rajas.

The concept provides the basis for one of the most individually creative and delicious meals ever. If you choose the right accompaniments, it can have an excellent nutrition profile. Because of the other items on the plate, as well as the way the steak is cut, the meat portion can be fairly small, 3½–4 ounces, yet still produce a satisfying meal. Bear in mind that a very lean 4-ounce tenderloin has about 120 calories, which allows another 280 calories if you are aiming at a meal totaling 450 calories—an amazingly low count for such a feast! One of my favorite versions is to add just an enchilada or two for steak and enchiladas. This also works nicely with the Grilled Top Sirloin.

Following is the recipe for the steak and calorie counts for recommended accompaniments, so you can pick whatever combination works for you.

INGREDIENTS

**4 (¼-pound) lean tenderloin steaks, preferably from the middle or
   small end, about 1¾–2 inches thick**
Juice from one lime
½ teaspoon kosher salt
Canola oil, as necessary

DIRECTIONS

Put one of the steaks on its side with the wide portion (normally the top or bottom of the steak) now becoming the side. Starting at the top, about ⅓-inch from one end, with a sharp boning knife, slice straight down, stopping about ⅓-inch from the bottom. Leaving the blade where it is, turn the steak so that the blade is once again at the high point, and once again cut toward—but not all the way to—the bottom. Keep doing this until you have basically unrolled the steak into one piece of meat about ⅓-inch thick. You can smooth out any uneven places by gently pounding the meat. Just before cooking, brush the meat with the lime juice and sprinkle on some salt. Repeat with the other steaks.

Either broil the steaks over very hot coals or sauté them on a very hot griddle or in a skillet with just a little oil.

Serve the steaks with one or more of the items in the list to the left.

PORK ENTRÉES

PORK IS MEXICO'S most popular meat, especially in the central and southern parts of the country. While many favorite pork dishes have too much fat and too many calories to fit into a healthy lifestyle, except, of course, as an occasional splurge, fortunately, many others offer considerable rewards without seriously compromising nutrition.

Puerco Estilo Vampiro

VAMPIRE'S PORK

4 servings

PER SERVING | 430 calories
49 g protein | 23 g carbohydrates
9 g total fat (2 g saturated)
145 mg cholesterol | 2 g fiber
15 g sugar | 420 mg sodium

In Mexico, tequila is often drunk with a chaser of sangrita, *which is made with a combination of orange juice, grenadine, chile, and sometimes tomato juice. When tequila is mixed with* sangrita *and topped with club soda, the cocktail is called a Vampiro. Those are the ingredients used in this delicious* alta cocina *offering, inspired by a recipe in* La cocina de Laura, *by Laura B. de Caraza Campos.*

INGREDIENTS

For the sauce

2 medium-sized ancho chiles, toasted and rehydrated (pages 15–16)
2 cups freshly squeezed orange juice
3 tablespoons freshly squeezed lime juice
¼ cup grenadine
½ cup silver tequila
½ teaspoon salt
1 teaspoon dried thyme
1 cup sliced white onion

2 pork tenderloins, about 1 pound each
1½ teaspoons pepper
2 tablespoons extra-virgin olive oil

DIRECTIONS

Preheat your oven to 350°F.

Make the sauce. Put the chiles in a blender with the orange juice, lime juice, grenadine, and tequila. Blend for 1 minute, or until the chiles are thoroughly puréed. Pour into a bowl, add the salt, thyme, and onions, and reserve.

Braise the pork. Season the pork tenderloins with the pepper. Heat the oil in a Dutch oven or similar heavy oven-safe pot over medium-high heat until it shimmers. Add the pork and brown all sides. Remove the pot from the heat, pour out a little of the oil, and add the chile sauce. Return the pot to the heat and cook on medium-high until the sauce just comes to a simmer. Place the pot in the oven and cook, uncovered, until the pork reaches 140°F, about 30 minutes, basting with the sauce every 10 minutes. Remove the pork to a cutting board, tent it loosely with foil, and allow it to rest for 5 minutes. While the meat is resting, reduce the sauce over high heat until it coats the back of a spoon.

To serve, slice the pork as thick or thin as you like, place it on serving plates, and spoon some of the sauce over the meat. White Mexican-style rice (page 61) goes particularly well with this dish.

Asado de Boda

WEDDING STEW

~~~~~~~~~~~~~~~~~~~~~~

4 servings

PER SERVING | 280 calories
37 g protein | 9 g carbohydrates
10 g total fat (2.5 g saturated)
110 mg cholesterol | 2 g fiber
2 g sugar | 560 mg sodium

Traditionally served at weddings in parts of northern Mexico, Asado de Boda is actually a very simple and exceptionally delicious mole. And it may be the inspiration for New Mexico's famous Carne Adovada. This recipe substitutes lean pork tenderloin for the more usual—and fatty—pork shoulder. The result is a great "reward" meal, where Splenda can be used effectively.

INGREDIENTS

1½ large or 2 medium ancho chiles, toasted and rehydrated (pages 15–16)

2¼ cups water

1½ tablespoons extra-virgin olive oil, plus more for browning the meat if necessary

1½ pounds pork tenderloin, cut into ½–¾-inch pieces

½ cup chopped white onion

3 cloves garlic, finely chopped

¼ teaspoon ground cumin

½ teaspoon dried leaf oregano

½ teaspoon dried marjoram

⅛ heaping teaspoon ground cloves

¼ heaping teaspoon cinnamon, preferably *canela*

2 teaspoons Splenda or sugar

¾ teaspoon salt

¼ teaspoon finely ground black pepper

1½ teaspoons cider vinegar

2 teaspoons finely chopped bittersweet chocolate

2 teaspoons finely grated orange zest

DIRECTIONS

Purée the chiles. Place the chiles in a blender, add the water, and blend to a smooth purée.

Brown the pork. Heat a pot over medium-high to high heat and add the olive oil. Stir in the meat and allow it to cook undisturbed until it is well browned on one side, about 30 seconds, then turn it to brown each side. When the meat is well browned on all sides, remove it to a bowl.

Finish the dish. Lower the heat to medium, add the onions to the pot, and cook, stirring often, until they are soft but not browned. Add the garlic and continue stirring until it is just cooked through. If you need more oil, add a little more olive oil or a spritz or two of cooking spray.

Return the meat to the pan, add the blended chiles and the remaining ingredients except the chocolate and orange zest. Bring to a boil, cover, and turn the heat down so that the liquid stays at a medium simmer and continue cooking for 50 minutes. Uncover the pot and raise the heat to bring the liquid to a brisk simmer. Cook until the sauce is thick enough to coat the meat. Stir in the chocolate and orange peel and simmer, stirring constantly, for 1 minute. Serve with hot corn tortillas.

Carnitas

4 servings

PER SERVING | 250 calories | 31 g protein 4 g carbohydrates | 12 g total fat (3 g saturated) | 95 mg cholesterol 0 g fiber | 3 g sugar | 390 mg sodium

I would never pretend that these are the traditional and beloved fried-in-lard carnitas. But they are not just a pale diet version of the succulent original either. They are more of a separate-but-equal choice—different but just as good in their own way. They make a tasty entrée and an excellent filling for tacos and enchiladas. Some of the milk is turned into little golden-brown cheese-like curds, which are one of the things that make it so delicious.

INGREDIENTS

2 tablespoons extra-virgin olive oil
1¼ pounds pork tenderloin, cut into ½–¾-inch pieces
1¾ cups whole milk
¼ cup orange juice
¾ teaspoon dried thyme
3 cloves garlic, finely chopped
½ teaspoon salt

DIRECTIONS

Preheat your oven to 325°F.

Brown the pork. Heat an ovenproof pot or Dutch oven over high heat and add 1 tablespoon olive oil and half the pork. Allow the pork to cook undisturbed until it is well browned on one side, about 30 seconds, then turn it to brown the remaining sides. When the pork has browned on all sides, remove it from the pot and repeat the process with the remaining olive oil and pork. When the second batch has browned, remove the pot from the heat, return the first batch of pork to the pot, and allow the contents to cool for about a minute.

Cook the carnitas. Add the remaining ingredients and stir until well mixed. Return the pot to the heat, bring it to a boil, and immediately put it in the oven. Cook for 1 hour, stirring every 20 minutes. Check periodically to make sure all the liquid has not evaporated. If it has, add just a little more milk.

Remove the pot from the oven, place it over medium heat, and bring it to a simmer. Continue cooking until all the liquid has evaporated and the ingredients—including the bits of cheese curd that will have formed—are a light golden brown. If all the liquid evaporates too soon in the oven, add just a little more milk. Serve the Carnitas with hot corn tortillas and Guacamole (page 59).

Tinga Poblana

PUEBLA-STYLE PORK STEW

This classic dish from Puebla is usually served with just tortillas, but it is also excellent with rice.

4 servings

PER SERVING | 370 calories
16 g protein | 29 g carbohydrates
16 g total fat (3 g saturated)
80 mg cholesterol | 9 g fiber
14 g sugar | 490 mg sodium

INGREDIENTS

1½ tablespoons extra-virgin olive oil
1 pound pork tenderloin, cut into ½-inch pieces
2 ounces homemade Mexican Chorizo (page 119)
1 cup diced white onion
1 garlic clove, finely chopped
1 (28-ounce) can diced fire-roasted tomatoes, with the juice
1 tablespoon finely chopped canned chipotle chile
1½ tablespoons adobo sauce from the chipotles
8 ounces carrots, peeled and cut into ½-inch pieces
½ teaspoon dried leaf oregano
¼ teaspoon dried thyme
¼ teaspoon dried marjoram
1 large avocado, chopped

DIRECTIONS

Sear the pork. Heat 1 tablespoon of the oil in a large pot or Dutch oven over medium-high to high heat until it shimmers, and brown the pork on all sides, 1–2 minutes. Remove the pork to a bowl.

Brown the chorizo. Reduce the heat to medium, add the chorizo, and cook, breaking it up, until it has cooked through.

Finish the stew. Add the remaining ½ tablespoon oil, the onions, and the garlic to the chorizo and continue to cook, stirring frequently, until the onions are soft. Add the browned pork and the remaining ingredients except the avocado. Lower the heat to a simmer, cover the pot, and cook 45–50 minutes. Serve the Tinga topped with the chopped avocado.

New Mexico–style Green Chile Stew

4 servings

PER SERVING | 350 calories
34 g protein | 16 g carbohydrates
15 g total fat (4 g saturated)
95 mg cholesterol | 3 g fiber
3 g sugar | 490 mg sodium

Green Chile Stew is one of New Mexico's most important culinary accomplishments. Made from pork, beef, or lamb, or all three, combined with the state's incomparable green chiles, the dish in all its many forms is a treat. In spite of using lower-fat ingredients, this version ranks near the top of the versions I've tried. The combination of pork tenderloin and lean ground beef allows both meats to become tender at the same time and provides a nice contrast of textures. There is no way to perfectly replicate the amazing flavor of New Mexico green chiles, especially those from Hatch, but blending a habanero chile with the broth brings the dish at least partway there. If you do not want the carbohydrates from the potatoes, you can replace them with carrots or hard tofu.

INGREDIENTS

3 cloves garlic, minced or put through a garlic press

1 teaspoon dried leaf oregano

¼ teaspoon ground cumin

2 tablespoons extra-virgin olive oil

⅔ cup chopped white onion

¾ pound pork tenderloin, cut into ½–¾-inch pieces

½ pound 96% lean ground sirloin

1 slice bacon, finely chopped

½ tablespoon all-purpose flour

½ cup chopped tomato

1 cup roasted, peeled, and chopped New Mexico green chiles, or
   substitute poblano or Anaheim chiles and 1 seeded habanero
   blended with the broth

2½ cups low-sodium chicken broth

½ teaspoon salt

1½ cups peeled and chopped white potatoes

DIRECTIONS

Make the seasoning paste. Grind the garlic, oregano, and cumin together in a *molcajete* or mortar and pestle and reserve.

Sear the onions. Heat a Dutch oven or similar-sized heavy pot over medium-high heat. Add ½ tablespoon of the oil and onions and stir-fry until the onions are soft and brown. Remove the onions and reserve.

Sear the meats. If you are not using New Mexico chiles, blend the seeded habanero with the broth and reserve it. Add the remaining 1½ tablespoons olive oil to the pot and add the pork. Allow the pork to sizzle until it is browned on the bottom, about 30 seconds, then stir-fry it until it has browned all over. Remove it from the pot and reserve. Lower the heat to medium and add the ground sirloin and bacon. Stir-fry, breaking the beef up with a spoon, until it has browned. Return the browned pork to the pot, stir in the flour, and continue to cook, stirring almost constantly for another minute.

▶▶

Finish the stew. Add the reserved garlic mixture, the tomato, green chiles, broth, and salt. Bring to a boil, cover the pot, and cook at a medium simmer for 30 minutes. Add the potatoes and cook, covered, for 20 minutes. Uncover the pot and continue simmering the stew until it is as thick as you like. If it becomes too thick, add a little more broth or water.

Carne Adovada

4 servings

PER SERVING | 340 calories
37 g protein | 11 g carbohydrates
14 g total fat (2.5 g saturated)
110 mg cholesterol | 1 g fiber
6 g sugar | 470 mg sodium

Carne Adovada is a classic and delicious northern New Mexico dish. It is another one that is rarely found elsewhere. It combines sweet, sour, hot, and salty tastes to produce a dish that is both bold and subtle. It is sometimes criticized because, traditionally it is baked without first browning the meat and onions, causing it to be less juicy and flavorful. This recipe cures that problem. It is important to use high-quality New Mexico chile powder (page 10). It is also important to let the meat marinate for 24 hours. In addition to an entrée, it makes a great filling for tacos and burritos.

INGREDIENTS

3 tablespoons extra-virgin olive oil
1½ cups chopped white onions
4 cloves garlic, chopped
1 teaspoon dried leaf oregano
3 tablespoons pure chile powder made from New Mexico chiles
½ teaspoon cinnamon, preferably *canela*
¾ teaspoon salt
1½ tablespoons rice vinegar
½ tablespoon agave nectar or honey
1½ pounds pork tenderloin, cut into ¾-inch pieces
½ cup water

DIRECTIONS

Make the seasoning paste. Put 1 tablespoon oil in a skillet over medium heat and add 1 cup of the onions. Cook them until they are caramelized to a golden brown, adjusting the heat as necessary to keep them from burning. Add the garlic and continue cooking until it is cooked through but not browned. Place the cooked onions and garlic in a food processor with the oregano, chile powder, cinnamon, salt, vinegar, and agave nectar and process to a smooth paste. If necessary, transfer the mixture to a *molcajete* and grind it until very smooth.

Marinate the meat. Put the pork and the remaining ½ cup onions in a nonreactive bowl. Massage the seasoning paste into the meat. Cover the bowl with plastic wrap and refrigerate for 24 hours.

Cook the meat. Preheat your oven to 325°F. Heat a Dutch oven or similar oven-safe pot over medium heat (400°F if you have a laser thermometer). Add 1 tablespoon olive oil and half of the marinated pork. Allow it to sizzle undisturbed until it is browned on the bottom, about 30 seconds, then stir-fry it until it is just browned on all sides. Remove the meat to a dish and repeat with the remaining pork. Combine all of the meat in the pot, add the water, and remove the pot from the heat. In order to thoroughly seal the pot, lay a sheet of aluminum foil over it and push the lid into it. Put the sealed pot in the oven and bake for 1 hour. Serve the Carne Adovada with rice or hot corn tortillas and Guacamole (page 59).

Grilled Pork in a Simple Fruit Mole

4 servings

PER SERVING | 300 calories
32 g protein | 22 g carbohydrates
9 g total fat (3 g saturated)
90 mg cholesterol | 2 g fiber
13 g sugar | 400 mg sodium

This mole *may be even easier to make than the Simple* Mole *recipe. I love the combination of prunes and dried mango, but the dish will work with nearly any dried fruit. Dried mango usually has added sugar, so if that is an issue, you might want to substitute something like apricots. I enjoy the pork either grilled entirely over medium-low coals or seared in a ridged grill pan and finished in the oven. The instructions are for the latter.*

INGREDIENTS

For the marinade and sauce
1 large ancho chile and 1 large *pasilla* chile, toasted and rehydrated, 1 cup soaking liquid reserved (pages 15–16)
1 tablespoon freshly squeezed lime juice
½ teaspoon dried leaf oregano
½ teaspoon salt
¼ teaspoon black pepper
1½ ounces dried mango, coarsely chopped
1½ ounces pitted prunes, coarsely chopped

1¼ pounds pork tenderloin
1 tablespoon extra-virgin olive oil
1½ cups chicken broth
1 teaspoon cider vinegar
2 tablespoons chopped dark chocolate or chocolate chips ▸▸

Make the marinade and sauce base. Put the chiles in a blender. Add the lime juice, oregano, salt, pepper, mango, prunes, and 1 cup of chile soaking liquid. Blend to a smooth purée.

Marinate the meat. Remove about ⅓ cup of the puréed marinade and sauce base and reserve the rest. Rub the ⅓ cup sauce base into the pork and refrigerate for at least 3 hours in a zipper bag or a nonreactive bowl, covered.

Make the sauce. Heat a medium-sized saucepan over medium heat, add the olive oil, and then stir in 1 cup of the reserved marinade and sauce base. Lower the heat and simmer, stirring nearly constantly, until it begins to thicken, about 5 minutes. Keep the heat fairly low or the sauce will spatter and make a mess. Stir in the chicken broth and vinegar, bring the sauce to a boil, and simmer until the *mole* is thick enough to coat the back of a spoon and is reduced to about 1 cup. Stir in the vinegar and chocolate, cook an additional minute, and remove the sauce from the heat.

Preheat your oven to 375°F and cook the meat. Heat a ridged grill pan over medium-high heat, add the marinated pork, and sear until well browned, about 1 minute on each side. Put the pan in the oven and roast the meat until it reaches 140°F, 12–17 minutes. Alternatively, you can grill the pork using the indirect-heat method.

Cut the pork into 1½-inch medallions, put them on serving plates, and top with the sauce. Serve with hot corn tortillas.

LAMB ENTRÉE

MANY MEXICAN lamb recipes, such as the various *barbacoas*, are made with fatty cuts. But the one offered below, originally from New Mexico, is a welcome exception.

Lamb Fajita-style

4 servings

PER SERVING | 350 calories
21 g protein | 8 g carbohydrates
26 g total fat (11 g saturated)
80 mg cholesterol | 4 g fiber
4 g sugar | 360 mg sodium

Some of the best lamb in the world is raised in New Mexico, and one of the foremost breeds, Navajo-Churro, is said to have been brought there by Spanish conquistadors. Years ago a friend in Española took me to a restaurant that featured lamb prepared fajita-style. It immediately became my favorite version of that dish, and I always serve it with the Chimichurri Sauce and a tomato-based salsa, Grilled Rajas, Guacamole, and flour or corn tortillas. To me, the marinade enhances the natural flavor of lamb, but feel free to omit it. The nutrition calculations are done with corn tortillas.

INGREDIENTS

For the marinade

1½ tablespoons tomato paste
5 cloves garlic, roughly chopped
¼ cup loosely packed fresh rosemary
1 teaspoon Worcestershire sauce
1 tablespoon pure New Mexico chile powder (page 10)
¼ teaspoon salt
½ teaspoon black pepper
1½ tablespoons freshly squeezed lime juice
½ cup canola or extra-virgin olive oil
½ tablespoon low-sodium soy sauce
½ tablespoon agave nectar
3 tablespoons chopped fresh mint leaves

1 pound lean part of leg of lamb, cut into ½-inch-thick slices
1 recipe Seared or Grilled Rajas, prepared without the lime juice (pages 70–71)
1 tablespoon freshly squeezed lime juice

DIRECTIONS

Make the marinade. Put all the marinade ingredients in a blender and purée. Marinate the lamb for at least 3 hours in a zipper bag or a nonreactive bowl, covered, if using the marinade.

Grill the lamb. Place the lamb over a very hot fire until it is barely rare. Allow it to rest 3–5 minutes, then slice it into bite-sized strips. This can be done well in advance, since the lamb will be reheated.

Finish the dish. Heat the Rajas in a skillet over medium heat. Add the lamb and cook until it is heated through and is either medium-rare or, if you prefer, medium. Add the lime juice and serve in the sizzling skillet or on a platter. For a real feast, serve with Chimichurri Sauce (page 51), Guacamole (page 59), and corn tortillas.

Naturally Healthy Mexican Cooking

SEAFOOD ENTRÉES

NUTRITIONISTS ARE unanimous in saying that we should eat as much seafood as possible. I believe they are correct because whenever I have eaten it nearly every day for at least two weeks, my bad cholesterol has dropped precipitously. The biggest problem is finding enough recipes that are delicious, quick, and easy for weeknight meals and that are different enough so eating them does not become boring. The recipes that follow solve those problems for me, and I hope they will do the same for you.

Pescado en Naranja

FISH IN ORANGE SAUCE

4 servings

PER SERVING | 360 calories
29 g protein | 15 g carbohydrates
21 g total fat (6 g saturated)
100 mg cholesterol | 2 g fiber
9 g sugar | 780 mg sodium

Veracruz was the first place in Mexico that Spanish settlers arrived. Many of the area's recipes, including the best known, Huachinango Veracruzana, are still close to their Spanish roots, with, of course, some Mexican twists. Fish in Orange Sauce is another delicious example. Originally made with butter, I think it is just as good with my favorite butter substitute, which has 40 percent fewer calories. It is also very quick and easy to prepare for a delicious weeknight dinner. You can use any mild fish fillet, including catfish. I adapted this recipe from one in the Gran libro de la cocina mexicana, *by Alicia and Jorge De'Angeli.*

INGREDIENTS

½ cup butter substitute
4 cloves garlic, peeled and smashed
1 cup minced white onion
1⅓ cups orange juice
4 (6-ounce) mild fish fillets, such as catfish
2 tablespoons pickled jalapeños, seeded, stemmed, and finely chopped
2 teaspoons pickled jalapeño juice
½ cup sliced black olives
1 tablespoon capers, drained and rinsed
½ teaspoon salt
1 tablespoon finely chopped parsley
2 teaspoons finely grated orange peel (from about 2 small oranges)
½ teaspoon black pepper

DIRECTIONS

Flavor the butter with garlic and cook the onions. Melt the butter substitute in a large skillet over medium heat. Add the garlic and fry slowly until it is soft but not at all browned; remove and discard the garlic. Add the onions and cook until they are soft but not browned.

Cook the fish. Add the orange juice to the skillet, and simmer gently for 2 minutes. Add the fish fillets and simmer until they are cooked through, turning once, 3–3½ minutes on each side.

Finish the sauce and serve. Remove the fish fillets to four serving plates, add the remaining ingredients to the pan, and simmer until the sauce has thickened, 2–4 minutes. Spoon the sauce over the fish fillets and serve. Sliced bananas make a great accompaniment.

Pescado Zarandeado

FISH ZARANDEADO

4 servings

PER SERVING | 250 calories
36 g protein | 7 g carbohydrates
8 g total fat (1.5 g saturated)
65 mg cholesterol | 1 g fiber
1 g sugar | 440 mg sodium

Pescado Zarandeado is a unique and delicious grilled fish dish served along Mexico's Pacific Coast, particularly in the state of Nayarit. Although it is usually made with snapper, you can use any fairly thin fish fillet, and I suggest you pick whatever one is freshest. In inland areas, that is often farm-raised catfish or tilapia. Some are surprised at the use of soy sauce, but it is a common ingredient in that part of Mexico, where many Chinese were brought to build the railroads in the early part of the twentieth century. The recipe illustrates the technique of brushing seafood with a little mayonnaise before grilling it, which produces great flavor and texture.

INGREDIENTS

For the garlic-chile paste
¼ cup extra-virgin olive oil
10 cloves garlic, minced
2 teaspoons annato seeds, ground to a powder
1 teaspoon low-sodium soy sauce
1 tablespoon pure ancho chile powder, or substitute New Mexico chile powder
¼ teaspoon powdered chile de árbol or cayenne
¼ heaping teaspoon salt

¼ cup mayonnaise
4 (6-ounce) red snapper fillets, or another type of fish
Lime wedges
Salsa of your choice

DIRECTIONS

Make the garlic-chile paste. Place the oil, garlic, and annato seeds in a small saucepan over medium-low heat and cook at a bare simmer until the garlic is just soft. Cooking it too long will make it rubbery and more difficult to grind into a paste. Lower the heat to very low, stir in the soy sauce, chile powders, and salt and continue to cook for 1–2 minutes, but do not allow the powders to burn, as they will be bitter. Remove the pan from the heat and let the mixture cool and the powdered spices rehydrate for about 20 minutes. Grind the mixture to a paste in a *molcajete* or mortar and pestle.

Flavor the mayonnaise and marinate the fish. Mix 1½ teaspoons of the garlic-chile paste with the mayonnaise and refrigerate. Spread a layer of the remaining paste on one side of each fish fillet (the nonskin side if the skin was left on) and refrigerate 1–3 hours.

Prepare the grill. Prepare a charcoal or wood-burning grill or a gas grill. Just before grilling, mix 1 heaping tablespoon of the flavored mayonnaise with the chives to use as a garnish for the finished dish. Spread the rest of the mayonnaise-chile mixture over the seasoning paste. ▶▶

Grill and garnish the fish. Grill the fish until well browned on the seasoned side, then turn and continue grilling until it is cooked through. Place the fish on serving plates, top with a little of the flavored mayonnaise and chives, and serve it with lime wedges, your favorite salsas, and hot corn tortillas.

Bagre en Adobo

CATFISH IN ADOBO SAUCE

4 servings

PER SERVING | 400 calories
29 g protein | 14 g carbohydrates
24 g total fat (4 g saturated)
100 mg cholesterol | 2 g fiber
7 g sugar | 370 mg sodium

This recipe is loosely adapted from one by Alicia and Jorge De'Angeli, two of Mexico's greatest food experts. The original recipe was designed for a whole catfish, but this one is for the more readily available and easier to use fillets. It has a terrific balance of sweet and savory chiles and mild vinegar. Besides being very good, it is also quick and easy to prepare and turns an easy-to-find, inexpensive fish into a great dining experience in no time at all. On the surface, it looks like it has a lot of fat, but it all comes from healthy olive oil, and much of it does not go into the finished dish.

INGREDIENTS

For the sauce
1 medium-size ancho chile, toasted and rehydrated (pages 15–16)
1 tablespoon chopped canned chipotle chile
⅔ cup water
⅓ cup rice vinegar
½ teaspoon dried thyme
½ teaspoon dried marjoram
½ teaspoon cinnamon, preferably *canela*
¼ teaspoon ground allspice
½ teaspoon salt

⅓ cup extra-virgin olive oil
3 cups sliced white onion, ¼-inch thick by 2 inches long
2 cloves garlic, peeled and coarsely chopped
Reserved sauce
4 (6-ounce) catfish fillets

DIRECTIONS

Make the sauce. Place the ancho and chipotle chile in a blender with the ⅔ cup water, the vinegar, thyme, marjoram, cinnamon, allspice, and salt. Blend for 1–2 minutes, or until thoroughly puréed, and reserve.

Cook the onions and fish and finish the dish. Heat a large nonstick skillet over medium to medium-high heat, add the olive oil and then the onions, and cook until the onions are becoming golden brown, turning down the heat as necessary to keep them from scorching, about 10 minutes. They don't need to be dark brown and caramelized, but they should be beginning to turn golden. Add the garlic and cook another 30 seconds. Add the reserved sauce from the blender, stir it into the onions, and add the fish. Spoon some of the sauce and onions over the fish and cook it, turning it once, until it is cooked through, about 3–3½ minutes on each side.

Serve. To serve, place a fish fillet on each of four plates and spoon some of the onions and sauce over each one. Accompany it with White Rice, or more simply, just some hot corn tortillas, sliced bananas, or fried plantain.

Aguachile Ceviche

WATER CHILE–STYLE CEVICHE

2 servings as an entrée, 4 as an appetizer. Nutrition information is for an entrée serving.

PER SERVING | 270 calories
30 g protein | 9 g carbohydrates
13 g total fat (2 g saturated)
45 mg cholesterol | 6 g fiber
1 g sugar | 200 mg sodium

Aguachile is a type of ceviche that is usually made with perfectly fresh raw shrimp placed on a plate and bathed with a purée of freshly squeezed lime juice, serrano chile, and salt. It is then topped with minced cilantro. Since finding shrimp of the proper freshness (sashimi quality) is often difficult in the United States, I tried making the dish with very fresh fish. The result was terrific! I added some chopped avocado and a drizzle of fruity extra-virgin olive oil to the mix, and it turned out to be perhaps the most refreshing ceviche I have ever had—and certainly the easiest to prepare. I have made it with fresh halibut, ahi, and even catfish. How long you leave the uncooked fish in the liquid will determine how "cooked" it will be. I prefer it left for only about 15–20 minutes.

If you want to use shrimp and are not sure they are perfectly fresh, for safety you can use regular shrimp that are boiled until they are just cooked through, and then put them in a bowl with ice and a little water to chill them as quickly as possible. You then put them in the lime mixture for about 15 minutes just before serving.

INGREDIENTS

⅔ cup freshly squeezed lime juice
1 medium-sized serrano chile (1–1½ coarsely chopped tablespoons)
½ teaspoon salt
½ pound sashimi-quality fish, or sashimi-quality or cooked and
    chilled shrimp
1 large avocado, chopped
4 teaspoons extra-virgin olive oil
Black pepper, to taste
Chopped cilantro ▸▸

Make the sauce. Combine the lime juice, chile, and salt in a blender and purée. Pour the purée into a nonreactive bowl and stir in the fish or shrimp. Refrigerate for 15–30 minutes, or up to 3 hours, depending on how "cooked" you want it.

Drain the fish, reserving the lime juice. Put the fish in a bowl, add the avocado, and toss.

For entrée portions, divide the fish and avocado into 2 portions. Spoon 1½ tablespoons of the reserved lime juice mixture over each serving and drizzle 2 teaspoons of olive oil onto each one. Season with pepper and garnish with cilantro. For appetizer portions, divide the fish among four small plates or large martini glasses, and portion the lime juice and olive oil appropriately.

Camarones Rancheros

RANCH-STYLE SHRIMP

4 servings

PER SERVING | 360 calories
21 g protein | 25 g carbohydrates
20 g total fat (3 g saturated)
145 mg cholesterol | 6 g fiber
13 g sugar | 550 mg sodium

One version or another of this dish is a staple up and down Mexico's Pacific Coast, and the following is one of the easiest and best. Instead of fresh tomatoes, the recipe calls for diced canned fire-roasted tomatoes. (Tomatoes are one of the few foods that are believed to be better for you when canned than fresh, because during the canning process beneficial lycopene is released from the plant's cell walls.) The amount of chiles given makes a dish that is medium-hot, so use more or less depending on your taste. Also be careful when adding salt because the tomatoes may have enough for the entire dish.

To quickly make a mild fish broth, simmer the shells and tails of the shrimp for about 15 minutes in 1¼ cups chicken broth combined with ¾ cup clam juice, or you can use plain chicken broth. It takes about 1½ pounds of frozen, unpeeled shrimp to make 1 pound after thawing and peeling.

As an entrée, the dish goes well with rice, but I like it served with only hot corn tortillas. It is also delicious in soft tacos.

INGREDIENTS

⅓ cup extra-virgin olive oil

4 large cloves garlic, smashed

2 cups finely chopped white onion

2 tablespoons finely chopped serrano chiles

2 (14½-ounce) cans diced fire-roasted tomatoes

1 teaspoon leaf oregano

2 cups fish or chicken broth (see above)

Salt, to taste

1 pound shrimp (21–25 per pound), weighed after thawing and peeling

Infuse the cooking oil with garlic. In a skillet heat the olive oil over medium heat until it shimmers. Add the garlic and cook until it just begins to brown, then discard it.

Sauté the onions. Add the onions and serrano to the skillet and sauté, stirring frequently, until the onions begin to turn golden brown. Do not allow them to fully brown as they can overpower the delicate shrimp.

Finish the dish. Add the tomatoes, oregano, and broth to the skillet, bring to a boil, and simmer until the sauce is thick enough to hold together and is no longer runny, 20–30 minutes. Add the shrimp and cook, stirring often, until they are just cooked through.

Pozole de Mariscos en Chile Rojo

SEAFOOD POZOLE WITH RED CHILE

4 servings. Nutrition calculations are made with homemade hominy.

PER SERVING | 340 calories
25 g protein | 37 g carbohydrates
11 g total fat (2 g saturated)
65 mg cholesterol | 3 g fiber
4 g sugar | 410 mg sodium

Although the traditional way to make this delicious pozole is with a seafood broth, for convenience it can also be made with chicken broth, vegetable broth, clam juice, or any of these fortified by simmering shrimp shells or fish trimmings in it for about 10 minutes. It can also be made with just about any seafood or a combination, including shrimp, crab, scallops, fish, whatever is freshest. In many places that is often catfish, which is farm-raised and therefore sustainable, and that is what was used in the nutrition calculations. Please do not try to save time by not roasting the onion and garlic, which adds a lot of flavor.

INGREDIENTS

4 large cloves garlic, unpeeled
1 (½-inch-thick) slice of white onion
4 guajillo chiles, toasted and rehydrated (pages 15–16)
3 cups low-sodium fish, chicken, or vegetable broth, or 2 cups chicken broth mixed with 1 cup clam juice
2 tablespoons extra-virgin olive oil
½ cup diced carrots
½ cup diced white onion
3 cups Home-cooked Hominy (page 76), or 2 (15½-ounce) cans hominy, drained
1 teaspoon dried leaf oregano
½ teaspoon salt, or to taste
½ teaspoon black pepper, or to taste
1 pound seafood, such as fish fillets cut to bite size, shrimp, crab, or scallops
1 tablespoon plus 1 teaspoon freshly squeezed lime juice
¼ cup loosely packed chopped cilantro
3 cups shredded iceberg lettuce
Lime wedges ▸▸

Roast the garlic and onion. Place the unpeeled garlic and the onion slice in an ungreased skillet over just over medium heat. Cook, turning from time to time, until the garlic skins are browned and the insides soft and the onion is very soft and somewhat browned, 6–10 minutes. Peel the garlic and put it and the onion in a blender.

Finish the cooking broth. Add the chiles and the broth and purée, about 2 minutes.

Finish the pozole. Heat a soup pot over medium heat, add the olive oil, carrots, and onion, and sauté until the onion is quite soft but not browned, 5–7 minutes, turning down the heat as necessary to prevent scorching. Stir in the hominy, oregano, and reserved chile broth, bring to a boil, and simmer gently for 15 minutes. Taste and add salt and pepper as needed. Stir in the seafood and continue simmering until it is cooked through, just a few minutes. Add the lime juice and cilantro.

Ladle the Pozole into soup bowls, top with lettuce, and serve with lime wedges.

Escabeche de Salmón con Mango y Aguacate

SALMON WITH MANGO-AVOCADO SALSA

4 servings

PER SERVING | 480 calories
41 g protein | 20 g carbohydrates
27 g total fat (4 g saturated)
100 mg cholesterol | 5 g fiber
11 g sugar | 600 mg sodium

You would have to be clairvoyant to realize how good this dish is just from reading the recipe. I adapted it after watching Chef Norman Van Aiken make Snapper Escabeche Tacos on Ming Tsai's cooking program. I added some ingredients and techniques from Mexico's escabeche tradition, substituted Jalisco's version of pico de gallo and avocado for the salsa, and converted the dish to an entrée. The result is perhaps the best salmon dish I have ever had—a real splurge with only healthy consequences!

The word escabeche *means "pickled" and when applied to seafood usually refers to fish that has been fried with a rub of fragrant spices then allowed to marinate in a solution that includes fruit juices and/or vinegar. You can skip the toasting and grinding of the cumin and peppercorns by using their ground versions, but if you can, please try the recipe as written.*

While the preparation requires three steps, they are all easy and reasonably quick and make enough for an entrée course without any side dishes. Each step is important and should be tried as written at least once before making omissions or substitutions. One final note: Nothing is more disappointing than overcooked fish, so err on the side of undercooking. As you will see, undercooking can be easily corrected before serving.

INGREDIENTS

For the spice rub

½ tablespoon whole cumin seeds or ground cumin

½ tablespoon whole peppercorns or ground pepper

¾ teaspoon sugar

¾ teaspoon kosher salt, or ½ teaspoon regular salt

¼ teaspoon ground allspice

¼ teaspoon cinnamon, preferably *canela*

¼ teaspoon ground cloves

For the escabeche

4 cloves garlic, finely chopped

⅔ cup very thinly sliced red onion

½ cup loosely packed chopped cilantro

3 tablespoons tequila

3 tablespoons sherry vinegar

3 tablespoons orange juice

1 tablespoon Valentina Salsa Picante or Crystal Louisiana-style Hot Sauce

1 tablespoon low-sodium soy sauce

For the mango-avocado salsa

1 large avocado, cut into ½-inch pieces

1½ cups Jalisco-style Pico de Gallo (page 38)

2 teaspoons extra-virgin olive oil

⅛ teaspoon salt

To finish

Reserved rub

4 fairly thin (6-ounce) salmon fillets, skins removed

3 tablespoons extra-virgin olive oil

Reserved escabeche

Reserved mango-avocado salsa

DIRECTIONS

Make the spice rub. If using the whole cuminseed and peppercorns, toast them in an ungreased skillet over medium heat until they are fragrant, 1–2 minutes, but do not allow them to scorch. Allow them to cool and then grind them to a powder in a spice or coffee grinder and combine with the other spices.

Make the escabeche. Combine all the escabeche ingredients and reserve.

Make the mango-avocado salsa. Combine all the salsa ingredients and reserve. ▶▶

To finish. Cover one side of each fillet with the rub and reserve, refrigerated, until ready to cook.

Heat a skillet over medium to medium-high heat, add the olive oil, and sauté the salmon, seasoned side down, until it is half done, about 2 minutes. Turn the salmon and continue sautéing for another 45 seconds to 1 minute, or until the salmon is still fairly rare.

Add the escabeche. Add the escabeche to the skillet. Simmer for about 15 seconds, remove the skillet from the heat, and allow the salmon to continue cooking and marinating in the residual heat for 3–5 minutes, spooning some of the sauce over the top several times. Just before serving, check the salmon for doneness. If you think it is underdone, reheat and cook it until it is to your liking.

Place each fillet on a plate, top with a tablespoon or 2 of the escabeche, then with the mango-avocado salsa.

Carnitas de Atún

TUNA CARNITAS

4 servings

PER SERVING | 300 calories
30 g protein | 25 g carbohydrates
8 g total fat (1 g saturated)
45 mg cholesterol | 4 g fiber
2 g sugar | 90 mg sodium

This dish is a perfect example of alta cocina mexicana. *Light and elegant but still earthy, this recipe is a delicious way to serve one of the world's healthiest foods. The recipe imitates the traditional preparation of fatty pork cooked in lard called* carnitas, *but uses much lighter ingredients and in a fraction of the time. When I saw it on Chef Rick Bayless's cooking show, I couldn't believe I hadn't thought of it myself. Deep-frying in oil with no batter or breading is the way that Puerto Nuevo's famous lobster dish is prepared (page 205), and I have been using that technique with more reasonably priced shrimp and scallops for years. Because of tuna's texture, it creates much the same crunchy exterior contrasted with a soft interior that makes pork Carnitas so popular. The fish takes on very little oil, making it a healthy and slimming dish, as well as delicious.*

INGREDIENTS

Canola oil for frying
1 pound ahi (yellowfin tuna), preferably sashimi quality, cut into
    pieces about 3 inches long, 1 inch wide, and ¾-inch thick
8 hot corn tortillas
½ cup Guacamole (page 59)
Salsa
Lime wedges

DIRECTIONS

Heat the oil and cook the fish. Put about 2 inches of oil in a fairly deep pot about 6 inches in diameter and heat it to 350°–375°F. Add the fish and cook for about 1 minute. At first, the pieces of fish will try to stick together in the oil, so keep them separated with kitchen tongs. They should be crispy brown on the outside and still a bit rare in the center.

Diners should cut their portions into bite-sized pieces, place them in a corn tortilla, and top with Guacamole, salsa, and a spritz of lime juice.

Salmón con Salsa de Granadas y Chipotle

SALMON WITH POMEGRANATE-CHIPOTLE REDUCTION

4 servings

PER SERVING | 320 calories
39 g protein | 15 g carbohydrates
11 g total fat (1.5 g saturated)
100 mg cholesterol | 0 g fiber
14 g sugar | 125 mg sodium

Nutrition experts suggest eating salmon more than once a week. I have found that if I want to have the same ingredient several times a week and continue to enjoy it, I need recipes that are both different and delicious. This alta cocina salmon dish is a favorite. It is so quick and easy that it is perfect for a weeknight meal, and it is so good that it's ideal for entertaining.

INGREDIENTS

For the pomegranate-chipotle reduction
½ cup pomegranate juice
½ cup balsamic vinegar
½ cup low-sodium chicken broth
4 teaspoons agave nectar or honey
1 teaspoon adobo sauce from canned chipotle chiles, or to taste
¼ teaspoon dried leaf thyme
1 teaspoon extra-virgin olive oil

4 (6-ounce) salmon fillets
¼ teaspoon salt
½ teaspoon pepper

DIRECTIONS

Make the reduction. In a saucepan combine the juice, vinegar, broth, agave nectar, adobo sauce, thyme, and oil and bring to a boil. Simmer until the liquid has reduced to the consistency of thin syrup. There should be about ¼–⅓ cup. As the reduction approaches that state, the number of bubbles will increase, and it will thicken quickly. Watch it very carefully and turn down the heat, if necessary, and stir constantly to keep it from scorching. Pour the reduced sauce into a small container, cover, and reserve.

Grill and serve the salmon. Season the salmon with salt and pepper and broil it on a grill or in a ridged grill pan until it is as done as you like it. Place one fillet on each of four plates and heat the sauce in a microwave. Spoon a tablespoon of it over each one. I particularly like this dish served with steamed zucchini or roasted broccoli.

Callo de Hacha con Salsa de Manzana y Aguacate

~~~~~~~~~~~~~~~~~~~~~~~~~~~~

4 servings

PER SERVING | 260 calories
19 g protein | 16 g carbohydrates
14 g total fat (2 g saturated)
35 mg cholesterol | 4 g fiber
5 g sugar | 440 mg sodium

This quick and easy recipe was adapted from one by Chef Carlos Fuenmayor and comes together very quickly. It is one of the reasons I always keep scallops in my freezer. The salsa is not only full of good things but also makes a perfectly delicious topping for many other kinds of seafood as well as for poultry and pork. It is also terrific as a salad when mixed with shrimp, crabmeat, or chicken.

INGREDIENTS

For the salsa

½ cup minced red onion
1 small clove garlic, minced
3 ounces (about ⅔ cup) cucumber, peeled, seeded, and cut into ¼-inch pieces
1 serrano chile, seeded and minced
2 tablespoons finely chopped cilantro
1 large avocado, cut into ⅓-inch pieces
1 cup diced, cored, and peeled apple
2 tablespoons freshly squeezed lime juice
¼ slightly heaping teaspoon salt
Fresh ground black pepper, to taste

2 tablespoons extra-virgin olive oil
1¼ pounds large sea scallops

DIRECTIONS

Make the salsa. Combine everything but the olive oil and scallops and reserve.

To finish. Heat a skillet over medium-high heat, add the olive oil, and sauté the scallops for about 1½ minutes on each side, or until just barely cooked through. Serve topped with the salsa.

Camarones al Mojo de Ajo Estilo Español

SPANISH-STYLE SHRIMP IN GARLIC SAUCE

4 servings

PER SERVING | 190 calories
16 g protein | 3 g carbohydrates
11 g total fat (2 g saturated)
145 mg cholesterol | 0 g fiber
0 g sugar | 190 mg sodium

Since falling in love with the Mexican version of Camarones al Mojo de Ajo, I try every similar recipe that looks interesting. The Spanish-style shrimp tapas recipe in Susan Spicer's Crescent City Cooking *has become a favorite. The following recipe was adapted from it, and it is so good that I look upon it more as a splurge than anything else. A number of side dishes work well, including rice and steamed squash, but I think the best one is a simple basket of hot corn tortillas to soak up the delicious gravy. Please note that sweet smoked paprika produces a terrific result that cannot be matched by regular paprika.*

INGREDIENTS

2 tablespoons extra-virgin olive oil
4 cloves garlic, thinly sliced
1½ pounds large (20–25 per pound) shrimp, peeled, deveined, tails removed, weighed after thawing and peeling (2 pounds before)
¾ teaspoon red pepper flakes, Aleppo pepper, if possible
½ teaspoon smoked sweet Spanish paprika
½ teaspoon dried leaf oregano
⅓ cup dry sherry
1½ tablespoons butter substitute
1½ tablespoons chopped fresh basil
Lime wedges

DIRECTIONS

Cook the garlic. Heat the oil over medium heat and cook the garlic until it just begins to turn golden. Remove it to absorbent towels with a slotted spoon and reserve.

Finish the dish. Add the shrimp to the skillet and sauté them for about 2 minutes, or until they are nearly cooked through. Add the red pepper flakes, paprika, oregano, and sherry and mix well. Return the garlic to the pan, swirl in the butter substitute and cook 1 more minute. Stir in the basil. Serve with hot corn tortillas or crusty bread and lime wedges. Two tortillas each will add about 100 calories to the dish.

Salmón de Coco

COCONUT SALMON

4 servings

PER SERVING | 250 calories
38 g protein | 2 g carbohydrates
10 g total fat (2 g saturated)
100 mg cholesterol | 0 g fiber
1 g sugar | 220 mg sodium

Coconut milk used to be a health and diet no-no. Like so many other things, that former condemnation has turned at least partially to praise. This tropical salmon dish uses coconut milk combined with achiote paste to create a very easy, very quick dish that delivers much more than the little effort required. One item that goes very well with it and takes very little extra time is zucchini. Just cut it into ½-inch strips, dip it into the marinade, and grill it, starting just before you grill the fish. The dish works very well in a ridged grill pan.

INGREDIENTS

For the marinade and sauce

1 cup lite coconut milk
2 tablespoons packaged achiote paste (page 6)
1½ tablespoons canned chipotle chile, seeds removed
¼ teaspoon salt
½ teaspoon black pepper
3 cloves garlic, minced
1 tablespoon minced fresh ginger

Reserved marinade
4 (6-ounce) salmon filets

DIRECTIONS

Make the marinade and sauce. Place all the ingredients except the salmon in a food processor or blender and purée.

Marinate the salmon. Reserve 2 tablespoons of the marinade for a sauce. Put the remaining marinade in a nonreactive container and add the salmon. Marinate, covered, for 3 hours.

Grill and serve the salmon. Remove the salmon from the marinade and grill it over hot coals, on a gas grill, or in a grill pan. Serve each salmon fillet topped with ½ tablespoon of the reserved marinade.

Callo de Hacha con Salsa de Aguacate y Trufas

4 servings

PER SERVING | 250 calories | 19 g protein
9 g carbohydrates | 3 g total fat
(0 g saturated) | 40 mg cholesterol
3 g fiber | 1 g sugar | 400 mg sodium

The elegant taste of truffles goes beautifully with both sea scallops and avocado. The best scallops are the ones that are dry-packed. For this recipe try to get large ones and do not overcook them, which is easy to do. The dish will be especially elegant if you put the sauce in a piping bag or cookie press with a fluted tip and use it to top the scallops.

INGREDIENTS

For the truffled avocado sauce

1 large avocado, about 6 ounces when peeled and seeded
1 tablespoon freshly squeezed lime juice
2 teaspoons good-quality white truffle oil
¼ teaspoon salt, plus more for seasoning the scallops
2½ tablespoons sour cream or Tofutti
½ tablespoon minced serrano chile
2 tablespoons finely chopped cilantro

1⅓ pounds sea scallops
Black pepper, to taste
1½ tablespoons extra-virgin olive oil

DIRECTIONS

Make the truffled avocado sauce. Combine the avocado, lime juice, truffle oil, ¼ teaspoon salt, sour cream, serrano, and cilantro in a food processor and process for 2 minutes. If possible, put the sauce in a piping bag with a fluted tip or a similar device.

Cook the scallops. Season the scallops with a little salt and pepper on both sides. Heat the oil in a skillet over medium-high heat until it shimmers. Add the scallops and sauté until golden brown on the first side, about a minute. Turn the scallops and cook on the other side until they are almost cooked through, about 1½ minutes per side, or less, for thin scallops. You want them to be the equivalent of a barely pink medium-rare. Anything more and they will become tough.

Divide the scallops among four plates and top each serving with about a half tablespoon of the sauce.

Jaiba Rellena

STUFFED CRAB

4 servings

PER SERVING | 200 calories
24 g protein | 13 g carbohydrates
5 g total fat (1 g saturated)
90 mg cholesterol | 1 g fiber
1 g sugar | 480 mg sodium

I found this dish in a seafood restaurant many years ago in Guaymas, where it was served as part of a seafood combination plate. It consists of two parts: the crab filling, and a topping of flavored bread crumbs. I like to bake and serve it in individual oven-proof plates shaped like shells, about 6 inches in diameter, but you may use any oven-safe plate or a ramekin of the right size. You can also make it in a casserole dish. You may use unseasoned packaged toasted bread crumbs, but it is just as good, and better for you, if you make the crumbs with whole wheat bread. Heat bread slices in a 300°F oven until they are thoroughly dried but not browned, then tear them into pieces and grind them into crumbs in a food processor. For an extra-crunchy crust, use panko.

INGREDIENTS

For the crab filling

2 large egg whites
2 teaspoons freshly squeezed lime juice
⅛ teaspoon cayenne
1 teaspoon Dijon mustard
1 teaspoon agave nectar or honey
1 pound top-quality lump crabmeat
1 tablespoon finely chopped fresh chives
1 tablespoon finely chopped cilantro
½ tablespoon finely chopped Mexican mint marigold or
    fresh tarragon, or 1 teaspoon dried tarragon
2 tablespoons all-purpose flour

For the topping

6 tablespoons unflavored toasted bread crumbs (see above)
1 tablespoon freshly squeezed lime juice
½ teaspoon Dijon mustard
1 tablespoon minced parsley
1 clove garlic, minced
1 tablespoon extra-virgin olive oil

DIRECTIONS

Make the crab filling. In a bowl, whisk the egg whites until they are light and airy, about 30 seconds, then whisk in the lime juice, cayenne, mustard, and agave nectar. Add the crabmeat to the bowl and toss carefully with the liquid, breaking it up as little as possible. Add the chives, cilantro, and Mexican mint marigold or tarragon. Toss carefully but well, then stir in the flour. Refrigerate for at least a half hour to let the flavors meld.

Make the topping. Combine all the topping ingredients in a bowl. Preheat your oven to 350°F.

Finish the dish. Mound equal portions of the filling onto four plates or dishes, as described above, or put it all in a casserole dish. Cover the crab with the topping and pat it gently into place. Bake 20 minutes, or until the topping begins to crisp and brown, but do not allow it to burn.

Salchicha de Pescado y Pepitas

FISH SAUSAGE WITH
PUMPKIN SEEDS

4 servings

PER SERVING | 310 calories | 28 g protein
12 g carbohydrates | 17 g total fat
(3.5 g saturated) | 115 mg cholesterol
2 g fiber | 1 g sugar | 440 mg sodium

This unconventional but delicious fish sausage is amazingly easy to make: You simply enclose the filling in plastic wrap and steam it. You can use whatever fish you like, or even scallops or shrimp. If you do not want to eat the sausages right after cooking, allow them to cool in their wrapping and refrigerate. Reheat in a steamer just until they are warm.

INGREDIENTS

¾ cup hulled pumpkin seeds
1 pound mild, fresh fish fillets
½ teaspoon salt
4 teaspoons minced serrano chile
¼ cup minced white onion
2 cloves garlic, minced
⅔ cup cooked Saffron Rice (page 62)
¾ teaspoon dried leaf oregano
¼ cup very finely chopped cilantro
1 tablespoon freshly squeezed lime juice
1 large egg, well beaten
Plastic wrap
Kitchen twine

DIRECTIONS

Prepare the pumpkin seeds. Heat a skillet over moderate heat. Add the pumpkin seeds and cook until most of them have popped. Coarsely chop ½ cup of the toasted seeds and grind the remaining ¼ cup in a spice or coffee grinder.

Prepare the fish sausage ingredients. Chop the fish into ⅛- to ¼-inch pieces. You can use a food processor, but it is easy to overprocess. Put all the pumpkin seeds in a bowl with the fish, add the remaining ingredients (except, of course, the plastic wrap), and mix thoroughly.

Wrap the fish sausages. Tear off a piece of plastic wrap about 1 foot long and place it on a work surface. Place enough of the sausage mixture in the center of the plastic wrap to form a sausage shape of about 1 inch in diameter and 6 inches long. Wrap the fish tightly in the plastic wrap, twist the ends, and tie them with kitchen twine to make a 6-inch-long sausage. Repeat with the remaining filling. ▸▸

Cook the sausages. Place the wrapped sausages in a steamer over boiling water, cover, and steam for 10 minutes. Remove the steamer from the heat and let it sit, covered, for 5 minutes before serving.

Arroz a la Tumbada

THROWN-TOGETHER RICE

4 servings

PER SERVING | 370 calories
20 g protein | 48 g carbohydrates
10 g total fat (1.5 g saturated)
50 mg cholesterol | 3 g fiber
5 g sugar | 570 mg sodium

This is a simple but very satisfying dish that Zarela Martínez in Zarela's Veracruz aptly describes as a cross between paella and risotto. Although my version uses some shortcuts, most notably with the tomato and broth, the dish has both authentic texture and taste and comes together quickly. I particularly like it with shrimp, scallops, and calamari, but just about any seafood in any combination will work. The nutrition calculations were done with catfish. Diabetics can steam the seafood separately and mix it with whatever quantity of rice fits their meal plan. The dish should be made with a medium-grain Spanish-style rice; my favorite is Goya's California Pearl Rice–Arroz Tipo Valenciano, and that is what the liquid measurements are based on. (Some Spanish rice requires more liquid.)

INGREDIENTS

1 cup crushed canned tomatoes, preferably fire-roasted
2 cloves garlic, roughly chopped
½ cup chopped white onion
2 tablespoons extra-virgin olive oil
1 cup medium-grain rice
1½ cups low-sodium chicken broth
1 cup clam juice
½ cup thinly sliced white onion
4 teaspoons minced stemmed, seeded, and chopped jalapeño pepper
½ teaspoon salt
¾ pound fish, scallops, crabmeat, calamari, or shrimp, or a
    combination, cut into bite-sized pieces
2 tablespoons minced parsley
Lime wedges

DIRECTIONS

Make the tomato purée. Put the tomatoes, garlic, and onion in a blender and purée. Reserve.

Fry the rice. Heat a medium-sized pot over medium heat, add the olive oil and rice, and cook, stirring almost constantly, until the rice begins to turn golden brown, about 4 minutes. Add the tomato purée, raise the heat to just above medium, and cook, stirring almost constantly, until most of the purée has evaporated and what remains is thick, about 6 minutes. It is all right if the rice is singed a bit in the process.

Steam the rice and seafood. Combine the chicken broth and clam juice. Add 2 cups to the rice along with the sliced onion, jalapeño, and salt. Raise the heat to high and, when the liquid comes to a boil, cover the pot and turn the heat to very low. Cook for 10 minutes and check the rice; it should be not quite tender and still a bit soupy. Add the seafood, replace the lid, and continue cooking for about 6 minutes. Remove the lid. If the seafood is cooked through, stir in just enough of the remaining broth to make the dish a little soupy. If the seafood is not quite done, cover the pot and cook a few more minutes, or until it is cooked through. Serve garnished with the parsley and accompanied with lime wedges.

Langosta (o Callo de Hacha) Estilo Puerto Nuevo

PUERTO NUEVO–STYLE LOBSTER (OR SCALLOPS)

4 servings

PER SERVING | 330 calories
20 g protein | 21 g carbohydrates
18 g total fat (3.5 g saturated)
35 mg cholesterol | 2 g fiber
1 g sugar | 530 mg sodium

Nutrition calculations include the scallops, butter substitute, salsa, and tortillas. Each serving of rice equals about 100 calories, a serving of beans about 80 calories, and the guacamole about 80 calories

Situated on the Pacific Coast of Baja California between Tijuana and Ensenada, the once-sleepy fishing village of Puerto Nuevo now consists mostly of bustling restaurants serving a very special lobster dish. The recipe is really for an entire meal rather than just the main item. The tail of the Pacific spiny lobster is deep-fried without batter or breading. The result is anything but greasy and produces lobster that is crispy on the outside and amazingly tender. It is served with refried beans, rice, guacamole, melted butter, a salsa, lime wedges, and paper-thin burrito-size flour tortillas. It is truly a feast! Unfortunately, it adds up to a fair number of calories. However, you can select one or two of the accompaniments, serve them all in very small portions, or just serve the recipe as written. By using small portions of the starchy items, the meal can fit nicely into most diet plans.

Because lobster is so expensive, I often make this recipe with large sea scallops, which are nearly as good. The dish can also be made with super-colossal shrimp. This dish is great for entertaining because everything except the seafood and guacamole can be prepared a day or two ahead. The seafood can be fried in a deep fryer or in about 2 inches of oil in a 9- to 10-inch pot.

INGREDIENTS

Canola oil
4 small to medium lobster tails, removed from their shells, or
    1¼ pounds large sea scallops
4 wooden skewers, if using lobster
1⅓ cups Mexican Rice (page 61) or Saffron Rice (optional, page 62)
1⅓ cup Refried Black or Pinto Beans (optional, page 67)
4 tablespoons butter substitute, melted
Guacamole (page 59)
Pasilla Chile Salsa (page 42)
4 very thin 7-inch-diameter flour tortillas
Lime wedges ▸▸

Cook the lobster or scallops. Heat the oil in a deep fryer to 380°F. If you're using a pan, heat at least 2 inches of oil to the same temperature. As you add the seafood, the temperature will drop, so try to keep it as close to 350°F as possible.

If using lobster, pierce each tail lengthwise down the center with a skewer to keep it from curling. Using kitchen tongs, place each lobster tail or scallop into the hot oil, hold it near the surface for a few seconds then let it drop and go on to the next one. Fry the seafood until it is just cooked through. Because the ingredients come in very different sizes and because heat sources vary, there is no way to give specific cooking times. I usually remove a piece from the oil from time to time and cut into it to gauge the progress. The exterior will usually be starting to brown when done.

Serve the meal. Divide the cooked seafood and some beans and rice among four plates. Serve the melted butter substitute, Guacamole, salsa, tortillas, and lime wedges family-style.

Pescado Pibil

"PIT"-COOKED FISH

4 servings

PER SERVING | 220 calories
29 g protein | 11 g carbohydrates
5 g total fat (1 g saturated)
100 mg cholesterol | 0 g fiber
1 g sugar | 75 mg sodium

The word pibil, *which means "pit" in the Mayan language, is attached to the names of dishes from Yucatán state that were traditionally cooked in the region's* barbacoa *pits. Today, most restaurants, even in Mexico, cook them in ovens. Because this dish, made with relatively thin fish fillets, cooks so quickly, it is delicious made on a grill or in ridged grill pan. You can use nearly any kind of fish. My favorites are red snapper, salmon, and catfish. You can use the following kicked-up purchased achiote paste or the one in the recipe for Yucatán Pit-style Chicken (page 163).*

INGREDIENTS

For the achiote paste
¼ **cup purchased achiote paste**
2 **cloves garlic, minced**
¼ **teaspoon ground cloves**
⅛ **teaspoon ground allspice**
½ **teaspoon dried leaf oregano**
About ¼ **cup sour orange juice, or 2 tablespoons freshly squeezed lime juice and 2 tablespoons fresh orange juice**

4 (6-ounce) **fish fillets, ½- to ¾-inch thick**
Banana leaves to cover both sides of each fish fillet
Aluminum foil
Salsa X'nipek (page 42) and/or Yucatán-style Tomato Salsa

DIRECTIONS

Make the achiote paste. Put the achiote paste, garlic, cloves, allspice, oregano, and half the juice in a *molcajete* or food processor and grind to a paste. Keep adding juice until the paste is just thin enough to spread easily but not so watery that it will not adhere to the fish.

Prepare the fish. Using the back of a soupspoon, coat both sides of the fillets with the achiote paste. Cut pieces of banana leaf the size of the fillets and use them to cover both sides of each one, with the shiny sides facing the fish. Wrap the fillets and banana leaves in several layers of foil.

Cook and serve the fish. Heat a grill or ridged grill pan to just over medium and put the packets of fish onto it. It is difficult to give precise times for grills with unknown heat levels, but thinner fillets usually take about 10 minutes, thicker ones, about 12 minutes.

To serve, place the packets on plates and allow diners to unwrap them. Serve with the salsa on the side. A half avocado and lime wedges make a great accompaniment.

Camarones al Mojo de Ajo a la Mexicana

MEXICAN-STYLE SHRIMP IN GARLIC SAUCE

4 servings

PER SERVING | 240 calories
17 g protein | 7 g carbohydrates
15 g total fat (2 g saturated)
145 mg cholesterol | 0 g fiber
0 g sugar | 320 mg sodium

This recipe can be made with shrimp of just about any size, but to me, the bigger, the better. I like to use the colossal (8–10 per pound) variety and serve 2 per person. Use the Ultimate Mojo de Ajo salsa in moderation for a quick and delicious low-calorie fried shrimp experience.

INGREDIENTS

1 pound very large shrimp, preferably 8–10 per pound,
    deveined, the tails left on
1 cup milk
¼ cup all-purpose flour
¼ teaspoon salt
¼ cup extra-virgin olive oil
¼ cup Ultimate Mojo de Ajo (page 44)
Lime wedges

DIRECTIONS

Coat the shrimp. About 20 minutes before you plan to cook the shrimp, dip them in the milk and put them in a small plastic bag (a grocery produce bag works well for this). Add the flour and salt and shake the bag vigorously to coat the shrimp. Remove the shrimp from the flour, shaking off any excess, and put it in the refrigerator for at least 15 minutes. ▶▶

Cook and serve the shrimp. Heat the oil in a skillet over moderate heat for very large shrimp or medium-high for smaller ones. The goal is to have the shrimp golden brown on both sides at the same time they are cooked through. When the oil reaches 350°F (when a drop of water immediately spatters), add the shrimp. Cook on the first side until golden, turn, and repeat. For the 8–10 per pound shrimp, it should take about 2 minutes on each side. If necessary, cut into the shrimp to make sure they are fully cooked. Serve the shrimp topped with a little sauce and lime wedges on the side.

Trucha Asada

GRILLED TROUT

4 servings

PER SERVING | 450 calories
45 g protein | 1 g carbohydrates
28 g total fat (6 g saturated)
135 mg cholesterol | 0 g fiber
0 g sugar | 500 mg sodium

I think there is no better fish than well-prepared trout. Although not widely known, several types of trout are native to Mexico, mostly in mountainous areas. Single trout fillets are usually too thin to grill properly unless you have a screaming-hot grill. But when you sandwich two fillets together, skin sides out, they are easy to cook over a gas or charcoal grill until the outside is golden brown and the inside is still moist and tender.

INGREDIENTS

For the flavored butter
¼ cup butter substitute
½ teaspoon Dijon mustard
1 teaspoon freshly squeezed lime or lemon juice
1 teaspoon adobo sauce from canned chipotle chiles, or
   substitute any hot sauce
1 teaspoon minced parsley
1 teaspoon minced cilantro
½ teaspoon minced fresh Mexican mint marigold or tarragon,
   or ¼ teaspoon dried tarragon
1 teaspoon minced chives

8 fillets from 4 trout, about 4 ounces each
2 tablespoons extra-virgin olive oil
1 teaspoon salt, or to taste
Black pepper, to taste
Lime wedges

DIRECTIONS

Make the flavored butter. Combine the butter substitute, mustard, lime juice, adobo sauce, parsley, cilantro, Mexican mint marigold, and chives and refrigerate until ready to serve.

Prepare the trout. Press the 2 fillets from each trout together with the flesh sides touching and the skins outside. Brush the skins with a little olive oil, sprinkle each side with a little salt and pepper, and set aside.

Grill the trout. Heat a charcoal or wood grill or a gas grill until very hot. Grill the trout on one side until golden brown, 3–5 minutes, and then turn and grill on the other side until the flesh is cooked through. Serve the trout topped with the flavored butter and lime wedges on the side.

Shrimp Adobo

4 servings

PER SERVING | 290 calories
23 g protein | 5 g carbohydrates
16 g total fat (2 g saturated)
215 mg cholesterol | 0 g fiber
0 g sugar | 540 mg sodium

This is one of my favorite recipes, and it fits nicely into a healthy diet. Besides making a great meal, especially when topped with avocado slices, it is ideal for cocktail parties and makes delicious tacos when the shrimp are cooked without their tails. The adobo rub can be made in a mini food processor, in a molcajete, or in a mortar and pestle. Although the recipe is very simple, there is one problem: pasilla chile powder is difficult to find in stores, although it is readily available on the Internet. I have tried using all ancho powder, and the result is not nearly as good. If you order pasilla powder, make sure you get the true pasilla rather than ancho powder, because anchos are often called pasillas *in California.*

It is also quite easy to make the powder yourself from the chiles, which are much more readily available. Just remove the stems and seeds from the chiles, put them in a 325°F oven until they are dry but not scorched, 3–5 minutes, allow them to cool and harden, and grind them in a coffee grinder.

INGREDIENTS

For the rub
4 cloves garlic, very finely chopped or put through a garlic press
½ teaspoon salt
1 teaspoon dried leaf oregano
3 tablespoons pure ancho chile powder
3 tablespoons pure pasilla chile powder
¼ cup cider vinegar

Reserved rub
1½ pounds (21–25 per pound) shrimp, cleaned, tails left on
    (or off for use in tacos)
¼ cup extra-virgin olive oil
¼ cup loosely packed chopped cilantro, divided
Lime wedges ▸▸

Make the rub. To make the rub in a *molcajete*, grind the garlic, add the salt and oregano, and continue grinding to a paste. Add the chile powders and vinegar and stir to make a paste. Or you could use a mini food processor to process the rub ingredients to a paste.

Coat and marinate the shrimp. Using rubber gloves if you are sensitive to chiles, work the rub into the shrimp until they are evenly coated. Refrigerate, covered, for at least 1 hour or up to 4 hours.

Cook the shrimp. Heat a large skillet over medium to medium-high heat and add half the olive oil and half the shrimp. Cook, turning the shrimp once, until they are *just* done, as overcooking will make them rubbery. Turn them individually with kitchen tongs to make sure they all get turned. When they are done, toss them with half the cilantro. Repeat the process with the rest of the oil, shrimp, and cilantro. Serve with lime wedges.

Camarones al Carbón

GRILLED SHRIMP

4 servings

PER SERVING | 190 calories
23 g protein | 3 g carbohydrates
9 g total fat (1 g saturated)
215 mg cholesterol | 0 g fiber
1 g sugar | 400 mg sodium

I like to serve this dish two ways: bold and hot, or a bit more refined! The difference between the two is the marinade. The recipe is versatile in that it can be served as an entrée with coleslaw or spinach, with rice, with Caesar Salad (page 96), or as a filling for tacos.

INGREDIENTS

For the bold and hot marinade
½ cup freshly squeezed lime juice
10 cloves garlic, coarsely chopped
1 tablespoon low-sodium soy sauce
1 teaspoon salt
1 teaspoon dried leaf oregano
½ teaspoon dried thyme
1 tablespoon agave nectar or honey
3 tablespoons chopped canned chipotle chiles

For the more-refined marinade
¼ cup freshly squeezed lime juice
1 teaspoon salt
½ teaspoon whole leaf oregano
½ tablespoon mild chile powder, such as that made from ancho chiles
⅔ cup extra-virgin olive oil

1½ pounds large shrimp (21–25 per pound), peeled and deveined
Reserved marinade
2 tablespoons extra-virgin olive oil (for bold and hot marinade)

Black pepper, to taste
Lime wedges

DIRECTIONS

Make the bold and hot marinade. Blend all the ingredients and reserve.

Make the more-refined marinade. In a bowl, whisk together the lime juice, salt, oregano, and chile powder, then slowly whisk in the olive oil.

Marinate the shrimp. For the bold and hot version, marinate the shrimp for 15 minutes, stir in 2 tablespoons olive oil, and marinate for another 15 minutes. For the more-refined version, marinate the shrimp for 1 hour.

Grill the shrimp. Season the marinated shrimp with pepper to taste and grill over a hot charcoal, wood, or gas fire until they are just cooked through, about 2 minutes on each side. Serve with the lime wedges.

Brochetas de Pez Espada

SWORDFISH SHISH KEBABS

4 servings

PER SERVING | 320 calories
24 g protein | 14 g carbohydrates
19 g total fat (2.5 g saturated)
75 mg cholesterol | 3 g fiber
7 g sugar | 250 mg sodium

This dish is so good that I often serve it on special occasions and recommend it to upscale restaurant clients. The fish is best when cooked over hardwood or charcoal with hardwood chips but will still be very good cooked on a gas grill or in a ridged grill pan. If you choose the latter method, make sure your skewers are short enough to fit inside the pan. The recipe also works with salmon. The hoja santa *can be omitted, but do try to find it as it adds a great deal to the dish—as does the plant to your garden!*

INGREDIENTS

⅓ cup freshly squeezed lime juice

1 tablespoon pure chile powder made from ancho or New Mexico chiles

1 teaspoon salt

3 cloves garlic, minced

1½ teaspoons dried leaf oregano

⅔ cup canola oil

1 pound swordfish, cut into 1¼-inch pieces

1 large poblano chile, or a bell pepper, stemmed, seeded, and cut into ¾-inch pieces

1 white onion, cut into ¾-inch pieces

4 small Roma tomatoes, cut into 3 pieces each

24 (2-inch) pieces of *hoja santa* (page 11)

4 shish kebab skewers

The marinated fish

Lime wedges ▸▸

Make the marinade and marinate the fish. Combine the lime juice, chile powder, salt, garlic, and oregano, then slowly whisk or stir in the oil until it is well combined. Pour the marinade over the fish in a nonreactive bowl and marinate, refrigerated, for 1–1½ hours, but no longer, or the lime juice will begin to "cook" the fish, as in ceviche.

Parboil the chiles and onions. So that the chile and onion pieces will not be only partially cooked when the fish is done, parboil them by immersing them in boiling water for about 5 seconds. Plunge them into cold water to stop the cooking, then drain and dry.

Prepare the skewers. Thread the ingredients on the skewers in roughly the following order: 1 piece pepper, 2 pieces onion, 1 piece tomato, 1 piece pepper, 2 pieces onion, 1 piece *hoja santa*, 2 pieces fish, 2 pieces onion, etc. Continue in the same order (or one you prefer).

Grill the shish kebabs. Light a wood or charcoal fire, start a gas grill, or put a grill pan on the stove to heat. Grill the shish kebabs, turning them as each side browns, until the fish is just cooked through. Serve with lime wedges, a half avocado, rice, or just hot tortillas.

Shrimp and Nopalitos

4 servings

PER SERVING | 280 calories
20 g protein | 17 g carbohydrates
15 g total fat (2 g saturated)
145 mg cholesterol | 4 g fiber
4 g sugar | 710 mg sodium

This recipe and the similar vegetarian one for cheese and nopalitos are just two examples of how delicious this healing vegetable can be. If, like so many others, you once tried nopal cactus paddles and were put off by the okra-like mucilaginous gunk they exuded, please give them another chance. The cooking technique advocated by Diana Kennedy and, more recently, Rick Bayless gets rid of every bit of it, leaving a delicious treat that can be eaten as an entrée or made into tacos. Actually, both at the same time, as I like them served with just steaming hot corn tortillas. Before making the dish, please review the information on nopalitos in the ingredients section (page 12).

INGREDIENTS

3 tablespoons extra-virgin olive oil

2 cups chopped white onions, ½-inch dice

4 cups nopalitos, about 1 pound, cleaned and cut into ½-inch dice

2 cups of the Chile Sauce recipe, made with guajillo chiles, if possible, but any of the others will do (page 45)

2 cups chopped fresh tomatoes

1 teaspoon dried leaf oregano

½ teaspoon salt

1 pound large (21–25 per pound) shrimp, shells and tails removed

3 tablespoons chopped cilantro

DIRECTIONS

Cook the onions and nopalitos. Heat the oil in a large pot or Dutch oven over medium heat. Add the onions and cook, stirring frequently, until they are just beginning to brown, about 5 minutes. Add the nopalitos, cover the pot, and continue cooking for 5 minutes. Uncover the pot. You will see that the nopalitos have released their viscous liquid. It will look like a mess, but don't panic. Raise the heat to medium-high and continue cooking, stirring almost constantly, until you see that the stuff is gone and the onions are turning a deeper brown. Another signal will be that the crackling and sizzling sound becomes louder. This usually takes 6–9 minutes.

Finish the dish. Lower the heat to medium, add the Chile Sauce, tomatoes, oregano, and salt, and bring to a simmer. Cover the pot, and continue cooking for 5 minutes. Add the shrimp and cook, stirring frequently, until they are just cooked through, 2–5 minutes, but do not overcook them. If you need to, check by cutting into a shrimp; when they are opaque, they are done. Stir in the cilantro and serve with hot corn tortillas.

VEGETARIAN ENTRÉES

FEW IN THE United States are aware of the emphasis that Mexican cuisine puts on vegetarian dishes. It should not be surprising because before the Spanish arrived, the people relied principally on vegetables. Today, most Mexican towns of any size have at least one vegetarian restaurant. However, Tex-Mex and other branches of Mexican American cooking, where most of our experience comes from, put little emphasis on vegetables.

Drinks

Low-calorie Cactus Smoothie
Atoles
Champurrado
Aguas Frescas
Horchata de Melón
Margarita
Sangría
Sangrita

Tortillas

Corn Tortillas
Flour Tortillas (made
    without animal fat)
Hybrid Tortillas (made
    without animal fat)

Salsas

Salsa Fresca
Salsa de Tomatillos Asados
Roasted-Tomato and
    Pumpkin Seed Salsa
Jalisco-style Pico de Gallo
Fresh Tomatillo Salsa
Salsa Ranchera
Mango Salsa
Salsa Habanero
Arizona-style Salsa
Pasilla Chile Salsa
Salsa X'nipek
Ancho and Chile de Árbol Salsa
Chile Pequín Salsa
The Ultimate Mojo de Ajo Sauce
Salsa de Chile
Cebollas en Escabeche
Pico de Gallo
Olive Salsa
Salsa de Molcajete
Yucatán-style Tomato Salsa
Romesco Sauce

Chimichurri Sauce
Cranberry-Jalapeño Jelly

Appetizers

Pickled Chiles and Vegetables
Hot Garlic Peanuts
Pepitas
Guacamole

Rice, Beans, and Other Side Dishes

Arroz a la Mexicana (use vegetable
    broth or water in place of
    chicken broth)
Saffron Rice (use vegetable broth or
    water in place of chicken broth)
Arroz Huérfano (use vegetable
    broth or water in place of chick-
    en broth and omit the ham)
Brown Rice
Frijoles de Olla
Frijoles Charros (made without
    the bacon and chorizo or with
    vegetarian substitutes)
Quick Beans
Santa Maria–style Beans (omit the
    bacon and ham or use vegetarian
    substitutes)
Refried Beans (made with olive oil)
Mexican Street Corn
Roasted-Garlic Sweet Potatoes
Sweet Potatoes Mashed with Coco-
    nut Milk and Roasted Garlic
Calabacitas
Seared Rajas
Caramelized Rajas
Grilled Rajas
Roasted Cauliflower
Roasted Carrots
Pozole Side Dish

Savory Corn Fritters
Calabacitas y Nopalitos
Grilled Prickly Pear Cactus
Quinoa

Soups

Sopa Tarasca (use vegetable broth or
water in place of chicken broth)
Caldo de Frijoles Negros (use vegetable broth in place of chicken
broth)
Caldo Tlapeño (use vegetable broth
in place of chicken broth and
tofu instead of chicken)
Gazpacho
Sopa de Lima (use vegetable broth
in place of chicken broth and
tofu instead of chicken)
Sopa Poblana (use vegetable broth
in place of chicken broth)

Salads

Ensalada Tequilero
Ensalada Caesar (omit the anchovy
paste and Worcestershire sauce)
Ensalada de Col

Egg Dishes

Tortilla Española
Huevos Tirados
Ojos de Buey
Chilaquiles Sencillos
Huevos Rancheros
Huevos Beneficiosos

Antojitos Mexicanos

Relleno de Hongos
Spinach Filling
Huitlacoche and Mushroom Filling
Tacos Potosinos (omit the chorizo)
Enchiladas Verdes (use cheese
instead of chicken filling)
Enchiladas Verdes Estilo Nuevo
México (use cheese instead of
carnitas filling)
Interior-style Enchiladas
Enfrijoladas
Sweet Potato Enchiladas
Enchiladas Sonorenses
(use olive oil)
Quesadillas de Elotes Asados y
Rajas
Mushroom Quesadillas
Spinach Quesadillas
Huitlacoche and Mushroom
Quesadillas
Tostadas (top with one of the
vegetarian fillings)
Gorditas de Papas (replace the
lard with butter substitute)
Cheese Crisps
Mexican Pizzas
Fresh Corn Tamales
Chiles Rellenos (made with one
of the vegetarian fillings)

Poultry

Pozole Verde (substitute hard tofu
cut into bite-sized pieces for the
turkey and vegetable broth for
the chicken broth)

Queso Panela y Hongos

PANELA CHEESE AND
MUSHROOMS, FILLING
OR STEW

~~~~~~~~~~~~~~~~~~~~~

*4 servings as a stew or
filling for antojitos*

PER SERVING | 210 calories
12 g protein | 21 g carbohydrates
10 g total fat (3.5 g saturated)
20 mg cholesterol | 4 g fiber
9 g sugar | 520 mg sodium

This dish is a reinterpretation of a recipe for a popular Mexico City appetizer served in upscale restaurants. In the original, a roasted tomatillo sauce is combined with panela *cheese, which is known for being slow to melt and relatively low in fat. They are poured into a fiery-hot* molcajete *and served with tortillas. In this version, sautéed mushrooms are added to the dish, producing a great stew and an outstanding vegetarian filling. It can be rolled in a hot corn tortilla for tacos or sandwiched between corn tortillas to make delicious flat enchiladas. The ingredients list may look a bit long, but the recipe is easily made in a few relatively quick steps and is well worth the trouble. As they say in Mexico, "Vale la pena." It can also be made a day or two in advance and reheated in a microwave oven. Panela cheese is widely available in supermarkets, and the only substitute I can think of—and it is not a great one—is low-fat string cheese.*

INGREDIENTS

¾ pound mushrooms, stems removed and cut into ½-inch dice
1 tablespoon extra-virgin olive oil
¼ cup minced shallots or white onion
1½ tablespoons minced parsley

For the tomatillo sauce
3 cloves garlic, unpeeled
¾ pound tomatillos, peeled and cut in half
2 tablespoons seeded and finely chopped serrano chiles
¾ teaspoon salt
¼ cup water

1 cup fresh corn kernels
Reserved tomatillo sauce
½ pound *panela* cheese, cut into ½- to ¾-inch pieces
Reserved mushrooms
¼ cup minced white onion
2 tablespoons loosely packed chopped cilantro

DIRECTIONS

Cook the mushrooms and shallots. Preheat your oven to 400°F. Toss the mushrooms with ½ tablespoon of the oil, spread them on a baking sheet, and roast them for 10 minutes. Allow them to cool. Drain and discard the liquid. Heat a skillet over medium to medium-high heat, add the remaining ½ tablespoon olive oil, and sauté the shallots or onions until they begin to brown. Stir in the mushrooms and sauté until they start to turn golden brown on each side. Stir in the parsley, remove the pan from the heat, and reserve. ▶▶

Make the tomatillo sauce. Heat a nonstick skillet over medium-high heat. Place the garlic and tomatillos, cut side down, in the pan and cook for 3–4 minutes, or until they are charred. Turn them and cook on the other side until they are soft, another 3–4 minutes. Place the tomatillos in a blender and peel and add the garlic when it is cool enough to handle. Add the chile, salt, and water and purée. Reserve.

Finish the dish. Heat a skillet over medium-high to high heat and add the corn. Cook, stirring often, until the corn browns and blisters a bit. Remove the pan from the heat.

Pour the reserved tomatillo sauce into a medium-sized saucepan and bring it to a simmer over medium heat. Add the cheese, bring the pan back to a simmer, and continue cooking for about 1½ minutes. Add the mushrooms and corn. Bring to a full boil and simmer for 1½ minutes. By this time the cheese should be melting but should still maintain its shape, and the liquid should be fairly thick. If not, continue simmering for another minute or two. Remove the pan from the heat and stir in the onion and cilantro. Serve with the hot tortillas, over rice, or as a dip with tortilla chips.

Guiso de Camotes y Ajos Asados

ROASTED SWEET POTATO
AND GARLIC STEW

4 servings

PER SERVING | 380 calories
5 g protein | 69 g carbohydrates
10 g total fat (1.5 g saturated)
0 mg cholesterol | 8 g fiber
32 g sugar | 540 mg sodium

This savory stew combines the recipes for Roasted Sweet Potatoes and Garlic with the sauce for Salmon with Pomegranate-Chipotle Reduction and a few other ingredients for a delicious vegetarian stew.

INGREDIENTS

¼ cup raisins
1½ tablespoons extra-virgin olive oil
2 cups chopped white onions
½ cup roasted, peeled, and chopped poblano chiles (page 16)
3 cups Roasted-Garlic Sweet Potatoes (page 73)
3 tablespoons Pomegranate-Chipotle Reduction (page 197)
4 ounces *queso fresco*, shredded
½ teaspoon black pepper
2 tablespoons minced cilantro

DIRECTIONS

Preheat your oven to 350°F.

Rehydrate the raisins. Put the raisins in a small container, cover with hot tap water, soak for 30 minutes, and discard the water.

Sauté the onions and chiles. Heat a skillet over medium-high heat, add the olive oil and onions, and sauté, stirring nearly constantly, until the onions are soft and beginning to char, lowering the heat if necessary to keep them from burning. Add the poblano chiles and continue cooking for a minute or 2. When the onions and chiles are done, put them into a medium-sized baking dish.

Make the stew. Stir in the sweet potatoes, raisins, Pomegranate-Chipotle Reduction, *queso fresco*, pepper, and cilantro and bake, covered, for 15 minutes.

Chiles Anchos Rellenos

STUFFED ANCHO CHILES

4 entrée servings, 8 as an appetizer

PER SERVING | 420 calories
10 g protein | 71 g carbohydrates
13 g total fat (2.5 g saturated)
5 mg cholesterol | 14 g fiber
15 g sugar | 650 mg sodium

While chiles rellenos are usually made from roasted and peeled poblano chiles, delicious versions are also made with ancho chiles, which are dried poblanos. This recipe includes a little tamarind, which you can make by rendering the paste from tamarind peels, but it is much easier to buy it in Asian markets already processed. Some tamarind pastes contain seeds, but you can dissolve the paste in the 2 cups hot water, strain, and discard the seeds and other roughage. I like to use both Roasted Carrots and Roasted Sweet Potatoes in the filling, but feel free to use one or the other. The chiles can be softened and the filling made a day in advance then brought to room temperature and assembled just before serving. The nutrition information includes an estimate of the amount of syrup or sugar left from the soaking liquid, but feel free to leave it out.

INGREDIENTS

For the chiles
1 tablespoon canola oil
2 cups thinly sliced white onion
3 cloves garlic, peeled and smashed
2 tablespoons tamarind paste dissolved in 2 cups hot water
1 cup *melao* (cane syrup) or brown sugar
½ teaspoon dried leaf oregano
½ teaspoon dried thyme
½ teaspoon salt
8 medium to large ancho chiles, slit down one side, seeds removed

For the filling
4 cups Roasted-Garlic Sweet Potatoes (page 73), Roasted Carrots (page 76), or a combination
2 ounces *queso fresco* or *panela* cheese, grated
1 teaspoon rice vinegar
Pinch salt
2 teaspoons extra-virgin olive oil
2 tablespoons grated *cotija* cheese ▸▸

Prepare the chiles. Heat the oil over low to medium heat in a medium-sized saucepan. Add the onion and cook until it has browned slightly. Add the garlic and cook another minute. Stir in the tamarind-flavored water, *melao*, oregano, thyme, and salt. Add the chiles, cover, and cook at a bare simmer for 10 minutes. Remove the pan from the heat, uncover, and cool for at least 10 minutes.

Make the filling. While the chiles are cooling, combine the sweet potatoes and/or carrots and *queso fresco* or *panela*. Whisk together the vinegar, salt, and oil and toss it with the vegetables.

Stuff and serve the chiles. Using a large slotted spoon, remove the chiles to a strainer and drain for 5 minutes. Carefully spoon about ¼ cup of the filling into each chile and put 2 on each of four plates. Spoon a little of the onions over each serving and top with the *cotija* cheese. Serve at room temperature.

Pasta Arriera

MULE DRIVER'S PASTA

4 servings

PER SERVING | 480 calories
14 g protein | 55 g carbohydrates
23 g total fat (6 g saturated)
10 mg cholesterol | 6 g fiber
3 g sugar | 210 mg sodium

This dish gets its name from the mule-driven transports that supplied Mexico with goods in the days before the train and automobile. Among other things, they disseminated cultural traditions, including recipes, from one region to another. I first had this dish, made with spaghetti, many years ago at the Hacienda del Sol restaurant in Juárez. It was fairly simple, and over time I made several additions. I specify dried orecchiette because that is my favorite for this dish, but you could use nearly any pasta. The portions of pasta may seem a little small, but I think you will find that when the other ingredients are added, the result is rewarding.

INGREDIENTS

For the sauce
2 tablespoons extra-virgin olive oil
3 tablespoons butter substitute
4 large cloves garlic, finely chopped
1 tablespoon seeded and finely chopped serrano chiles
3 tablespoons finely chopped sun-dried tomatoes (not the kind packed in oil)
1 tablespoon finely chopped ancho chiles
½ teaspoon dried leaf oregano
¼ teaspoon dried thyme
¼ heaping teaspoon salt
¼ teaspoon ground black pepper

To finish

9 ounces dried orecchiette pasta, or any other dried pasta

¼ cup grated *queso fresco*

¼ cup grated part skim milk mozzarella

2 tablespoons grated *cotija* cheese

2 tablespoons minced parsley

2 tablespoons minced cilantro

1 large avocado, chopped

Lime wedges

DIRECTIONS

Make the sauce. Heat the olive oil and butter substitute over just under medium heat until the butter substitute is melted. Add the garlic and serrano and sauté until the garlic is just soft but not browned. Stir in the sun-dried tomatoes, ancho chiles, oregano, thyme, salt, and pepper, and allow the pan to sit off the heat for at least 30 minutes.

 Finish the dish and serve. Cook the pasta until al dente. Pour it into a strainer and shake to make sure all the liquid is drained. Off the heat, return the pasta to the pot, toss with the sauce, cheeses, parsley, and cilantro, and divide among four serving plates. Top the pasta with the avocado and serve with the lime wedges.

Nopal Stew

4 servings

PER SERVING | 250 calories
11 g protein | 16 g carbohydrates
16 g total fat (5 g saturated)
15 mg cholesterol | 5 g fiber
7 g sugar | 520 mg sodium

This is the vegetarian cousin of the recipe for Shrimp and Nopalitos. It is at least as good and makes a delicious and nutritious meal. Panela cheese resists melting, and that is why it is used, so serve the dish when the cheese is warmed through.

INGREDIENTS

3 tablespoons extra-virgin olive oil

2 cups chopped white onion

2 cups chopped mushrooms

4 cups nopalitos, about 1 pound, cleaned and cut into ½-inch dice (page 12)

2 cups Chile Sauce (page 45), made with guajillo chiles if possible, but any of the others will do

2 cups chopped fresh tomatoes

1 teaspoon dried leaf oregano

½ teaspoon salt

4 ounces panela cheese, cut into ½-inch chunks

3 tablespoons chopped cilantro ▸▸

Cook the vegetables. Heat the oil in a large pot or Dutch oven over medium heat. Add the onions and cook, stirring frequently, until they are just beginning to brown, about 5 minutes. Add the mushrooms and continue cooking, stirring often, for 3 minutes. Add the chopped nopalitos, cover the pot, and continue cooking for 5 minutes. Uncover the pot. The nopalitos will have released their viscous liquid, and there will also be some liquid from the mushrooms. Raise the heat to medium-high and continue cooking, uncovered, stirring almost constantly, until all the liquid is gone and the onions are continuing to brown. The crackling and sizzling sound will increase as the liquid boils off. This usually takes about 6–9 minutes.

Finish the dish. Stir in the Chile Sauce, tomatoes, oregano, and salt, cover the pot, and continue cooking for 5 minutes. Remove the lid, add the cheese, and cook, stirring frequently, until the cheese is warmed and just beginning to melt. Stir in the cilantro and serve immediately with hot corn tortillas.

Papadzules

4 servings

PER SERVING | 520 calories
21 g protein | 35 g carbohydrates
35 g total fat (7 g saturated)
185 mg cholesterol | 7 g fiber
7 g sugar | 380 mg sodium

So unusual is this traditional dish from Mexico's Yucatán state that it is difficult to categorize, although it's probably closest to being an enchilada. No literal description can do it justice, so please trust me when I say that it is one of the most delicious foods there is. Although at 520 calories per serving, the dish is not as slimming as most others in the book, over 200 of those calories come from pumpkin seeds, which, with large quantities of omega-3 fatty acids, are a nutritional superfood. And the recipe makes a complete meal with no need for side dishes.

I have taken a few mild liberties to make the preparation easier, but I do not believe they change the outcome in any material way. For example, cooks traditionally extract the pumpkin seed oil by squeezing the seed paste, something that is time consuming and often only partially successful. Since pumpkin seed oil is readily available, it is much easier to just use a few teaspoons of it.

INGREDIENTS

7 ounces (about 1⅓ cups) hulled green pumpkin seeds

⅛ teaspoon salt

1 recipe Yucatán-style Tomato Salsa (page 49), tomato cooking liquid reserved

8 corn tortillas, softened with cooking spray (page 17)

4 large hard-boiled eggs, coarsely chopped

4 teaspoons pumpkin seed oil

DIRECTIONS

Toast the pumpkin seeds and make the paste. Heat a nonstick skillet over medium to medium-high heat, add the pumpkin seeds, and toast, stirring frequently, until most of them have popped, 2–3 minutes. While they are still hot, grind the seeds to a powder in a coffee or spice grinder and put the powder into a bowl with the salt. Add enough of the reserved tomato cooking liquid to make a medium-thick paste, about ⅔ cup. It should be easy to spread but not too runny. If it thickens before you use it, add more liquid.

Make the papadzules. Bring the Tomato Salsa to a simmer and hold while making the Papadzules. Place 2 hot tortillas each on four plates. Spread the tortillas with a thin layer of pumpkin seed paste. Divide the hard-boiled egg equally among the tortillas and roll as for enchiladas. Spread more of the paste over the rolled Papadzules. Pour the Tomato Salsa down the middle of the papadzules, leaving about 1½ inches at each end covered with only the pumpkin seed paste. Drizzle 1 teaspoon of the pumpkin seed oil over each serving.

Mushrooms Stuffed with Huitlacoche

4 entrée servings, 15 as an appetizer

PER SERVING | 45 calories
3 g protein | 2 g carbohydrates
3 g total fat (1 g saturated)
5 mg cholesterol | 1 g fiber
1 g sugar | 95 mg sodium

This dish uses the exotic flavor and texture of huitlacoche in a very simple way to great effect. It can be made as an entrée with large portobello mushrooms or as an appetizer using medium-sized button mushrooms. Nutrition amounts are for one small stuffed mushroom; the entrée analysis can be calculated by multiplying the numbers here by 7.5.

INGREDIENTS

**4 very large portobello mushrooms, gills removed, or about
    30 medium-sized button mushrooms**
Cooking spray
1 recipe Huitlacoche and Mushroom Filling (page 124)
⅓ cup grated *cotija* cheese

DIRECTIONS

Preheat your oven to 375°F.

Fill the mushrooms. Spray the outside of the mushroom caps with cooking spray. For the portobellos, spoon about 4 ounces of filling into each one and top with an equal amount of the cheese. For the button mushrooms, spoon about ½ ounce of the filling into each one and top with about ½ teaspoon of the cheese.

Bake the mushrooms. Bake the mushrooms on a baking sheet for 15–20 minutes, or until they are soft but not falling apart and the cheese is melted.

Breakfast Corn Cakes

4 servings, 2 fritters each

PER SERVING | 370 calories | 8 g protein
55 g carbohydrates | 14 g total fat
(4 g saturated) | 96 mg cholesterol
3 g fiber | 28 g sugar | 430 mg sodium

Just south of Monterrey, during its fiesta, food stalls in the town of Santiago serve the most delicious corn cakes I have ever had. The only problem is that, like fresh corn tamales, they are made from high-starch field corn rather than the sweet corn found in our markets. They also come with a fair amount of sugar. In an effort to re-create them with sweet corn and very little sugar, I modified Jacques Pépin's recipe for corn fritters. While my adaptation is slightly different in texture from the Mexican version, the general effect is so similar and so good that I decided to include the recipe in two versions: Breakfast Corn Cakes, and Savory Corn Fritters (page 77). Thinking that using dried corn flour instead of all-purpose flour would enhance the corn flavor, I tried it and was surprised at how little difference it made. In fact, both tasters liked it less than the one with all-purpose flour. In a pinch, the dish can be made with thawed and dried frozen corn.

INGREDIENTS

½ cup all-purpose flour
3 tablespoons cornstarch
1 teaspoon baking powder
¼ teaspoon salt
½ teaspoon grated nutmeg
2 large eggs, beaten
½ cup cold water
4 teaspoons agave nectar, plus extra for serving
3 cups fresh corn kernels, from about 4 medium-sized ears
6 tablespoons butter substitute

DIRECTIONS

Make the batter. Mix together the flour, cornstarch, baking powder, salt, and nutmeg. Beat the eggs, cold water, and agave nectar together and stir it into the dry mixture just until combined. Finely chop the corn or process it until finely chopped, but do not purée it, as it should still have some texture. Stir it into the batter and allow it to sit for 15–20 minutes to make sure the flour is completely hydrated and to allow the gluten to relax.

Preheat your oven to 150°F. Heat a large nonstick skillet over medium heat (350–375°F) and add 2 tablespoons of the butter substitute. Scoop 4 slightly heaping ⅓-cup measures of the batter into the skillet and pat them flat with a spatula. Cook the cakes until they are golden brown on the bottom, about 3 minutes. Turn the cakes and cook them until they are browned on the other side, about another 3 minutes. Put them in the oven to keep them warm while you make the remaining 4 cakes. Serve the cakes topped with the remaining butter substitute and agave nectar.

Rosemary Roasted Potatoes with Black Beans and Avocado

4 servings

PER SERVING | 450 calories
14 g protein | 41 g carbohydrates
27 g total fat (8 g saturated)
25 mg cholesterol | 10 g fiber
6 g sugar | 400 mg sodium

I do not know if this dish originated in Mexico or exactly what to call it except "my favorite vegetarian meal." I found it in a terrific vegetarian restaurant in La Jolla, California, called (oddly enough) The Coffee Cup. I use this version (which to me is very similar to the original) for everything from brunch to supper, and it never fails to delight. The best way to seed and devein the jalapeños is, wearing gloves, to cut them in half and scoop the seeds and veins out with a small spoon.

INGREDIENTS

¼ cup extra-virgin olive oil

3 cloves garlic, unpeeled

3 tablespoons fresh rosemary leaves

⅔ cup water

Scant ¼ teaspoon salt

12 ounces russet or Yukon gold potatoes, cut into ¾-inch pieces and thoroughly rinsed to remove the starch

2 jalapeño chiles, seeds and veins removed, cut into ⅛-inch-thick rounds

1 cup cooked and rinsed black beans

2 Roma tomatoes, chopped into ½-inch pieces

1 cup frozen corn kernels, thawed (measured after thawing)

1 large avocado, cut into ½-inch pieces

¼ cup finely chopped cilantro

¾ cup shredded, part skim milk mozzarella cheese

2 tablespoons hot sauce, such as sriracha

¼ cup sour cream or Tofutti

DIRECTIONS

Make the flavored oil. Put the oil, garlic, and rosemary in a microwave-safe container and microwave for 30 seconds on High. Wait 15 seconds and repeat. Allow the dish to sit, covered, at room temperature for 2–3 hours, and then strain the oil into another dish, discarding the garlic and rosemary. Stir in the water and salt and reserve.

Roast the potatoes. Preheat your oven to 425°F. Place the potatoes in a 9-inch cast iron skillet or similar oven-safe dish, add the oil-water mixture, and bring to a simmer over medium-high heat. Put the skillet in the oven for 30 minutes. Remove from the oven, add the jalapeño rounds, turn the potatoes, and roast for an additional 15 minutes, or until the potatoes are a crusty golden brown.

Mix the vegetables. While the potatoes are roasting, in a bowl combine the black beans, tomatoes, corn, avocado, and cilantro, and reserve.

Finish the dish. Divide the potatoes among four plates, top with equal portions of the vegetable mixture, and garnish with the cheese, hot sauce, and sour cream or Tofutti.

DESSERTS

MOST OF THE better known Mexican desserts are, unfortunately, filled with fat and sugar, except, of course, fresh fruits, which are very popular for everyday use. For this section I found some much healthier but still delicious alternatives.

Mousse de Chocolate

DAIRY-FREE CHOCOLATE MOUSSE

About 10 quarter-cup servings

PER SERVING | 130 calories | 4 g protein | 11 g carbohydrates | 7 g total fat (3.5 g saturated) | 0 mg cholesterol 2 g fiber | 8 g sugar | 45 mg sodium

Chocolate is one of Mexico's gifts to the world, and history records that the Emperor Montezuma often took his chocolate drink flavored with chile. When serving the following recipe, I often ask people to guess at the ingredients other than chocolate. Heavy cream is invariably at the top of everyone's list. Then I watch their jaws drop when I tell them that it is made largely from tofu. Try it and you will understand their surprise. I know it's hard to believe, but this is simply one of the best chocolate dishes I have ever had, and it is certainly the best for you and easiest to prepare.

One of the things that makes it so good is that, while its taste and consistency are light compared, for example, to ice cream, it is actually dense with chocolate. And that is good because nutrition experts now extol the virtues of high-cacao-content chocolate. Therefore, I have set the serving size at ¼ cup. For me, this amount, which includes the equivalent of one-sixth of a chocolate bar, is sufficient, especially when served topped with the Fruit Compote (page 228). If you do not want to use a liqueur, replace it with orange juice. It will still be good, just not quite as exotic. It is also terrific scooped into ice cream cones. Please note that the percentage of cacao in the chocolate you use is very important. For example, if you use only 40 percent cacao content, you will need to nearly double the amount you use to get the same consistency and flavor balance.

INGREDIENTS

1 pound silken or soft tofu
1 teaspoon vanilla extract
1 tablespoon honey
¾ teaspoon pure ancho chile powder
⅛ teaspoon salt
¼ heaping teaspoon cinnamon, preferably *canela*
5¼ ounces (about 1 cup) 70% cocoa dark chocolate cut into very small pieces
3 tablespoons Kahlúa, Grand Marnier, Cointreau, or triple sec, or substitute orange juice

DIRECTIONS

Put the tofu, vanilla, honey, chile powder, salt, and cinnamon in the bowl of a food processor fitted with the steel blade. Place a stainless steel bowl over a small to medium-sized pot of simmering water. Add the chocolate and liqueur or orange juice to the pot and stir frequently with a wooden spoon until the chocolate has completely melted, 1–2 minutes. Add the chocolate mixture to the food processor and process with the other ingredients for 1 minute, stopping as necessary to scrape down the sides of the bowl. Pour the mixture into a large bowl or into separate small serving dishes. Cover with plastic wrap and chill for several hours.

Compota de Frutas

FRUIT COMPOTE

4 servings

PER SERVING | 160 calories | 2 g protein
27 g carbohydrates | 0 g total fat
(0 g saturated) | 0 mg cholesterol
3 g fiber | 21 g sugar | 0 mg sodium

This dessert is a favorite for its exotic flavor and ease of preparation. Although it is delicious by itself, it is superb spooned over the Chocolate Mousse (page 227). It can be made with just about any kind of berry or other fruit, but my favorite combination is dried cherries and fresh blackberries. It keeps well for about a week, refrigerated.

INGREDIENTS

½ cup dried cherries
1 cup fresh blackberries
½ cup crème de cassis

DIRECTIONS

Mix all the ingredients together and refrigerate for 3 hours or overnight.

Bananas and Mandarin Oranges with Vanilla Sauce

4 quarter-cup servings

PER SERVING | 230 calories | 5 g protein
47 g carbohydrates | 4 g total fat
(1 g saturated) | 0 mg cholesterol
4 g fiber | 29 g sugar | 210 mg sodium

This delightful dessert introduces a delicious vanilla sauce made with soy milk that has many uses.

INGREDIENTS

For the custard sauce
2 tablespoons cornstarch
¼ teaspoon cinnamon, preferably *canela*
2 cups vanilla-flavored soy milk
1 tablespoon butter substitute
2 tablespoons agave nectar
½ teaspoon vanilla extract
¼ teaspoon salt

To finish
3 cups diced bananas
1 cup drained canned mandarin oranges

DIRECTIONS

Make the custard sauce. Put the cornstarch and cinnamon in a small saucepan and stir in the soy milk a tablespoon or 2 at a time until well combined. Stir in the rest of the milk in a thin stream and add the butter substitute. Bring to a boil and simmer until it thickens to the consistency of light custard, about 10 minutes. Stir in agave nectar, vanilla, salt, and remove from heat.

Finish the dessert. Allow the sauce to cool slightly and pour it over the cut-up fruit.

Sorbete de Jamaica

HIBISCUS PETAL SORBET

~~~~~~~~~~~~~~~~~~~~~~~

5 half-cup servings

PER SERVING | 180 calories | 0 g protein
43 g carbohydrates | 0 g total fat
(0 g saturated) | 0 mg cholesterol
0 g fiber | 42 g sugar | 0 mg sodium

Called jamaica *in Spanish, the petals of the hibiscus flower are dried and made into a tea that is sweetened to produce a popular soft drink throughout Mexico. Hibiscus tea also makes a refreshing sorbet. You can omit the limoncello, but that or another liqueur is important because it helps keep the sorbet from freezing into a solid block of ice.*

INGREDIENTS

2½ cups dried *jamaica* leaves (available at Hispanic groceries)
1 quart water
½ ounce fresh ginger, finely chopped
1 cup sugar
1 tablespoon freshly squeezed lime juice
2 tablespoons limoncello

DIRECTIONS

Make the tea. Place the *jamaica* leaves in a pot or bowl, bring the water to a boil, and pour it over the leaves. Cover and steep for 15 minutes. Strain the tea and discard the *jamaica*.

Make the sorbet base. Put the ginger in a blender, add 1 cup of the tea, and blend until completely puréed, 1–2 minutes. Add another 1½ cups of tea and blend again.

Pour the sorbet base into a pot, add the sugar, and bring to a boil, stirring to dissolve the sugar. Remove the pot from the heat as soon as the sorbet base comes to a boil. Stir in the lime juice and cool. Refrigerate the base until it reaches 60°F.

Freeze the sorbet. Add the limoncello to the chilled base and pour it into an ice cream maker. Freeze according to the manufacturer's directions until it is frozen but still slushy, 20–30 minutes.

Grilled Mangoes

4 servings

PER SERVING | 130 calories | 2 g protein
34 g carbohydrates | 0 g total fat
(0 g saturated) | 0 mg cholesterol
3 g fiber | 31 g sugar | 0 mg sodium

The idea for this casual but terrific desert came from Bobby Flay, whose San Antonio show was filmed in my outdoor kitchen. Mangoes are grilled briefly to create grill marks, which provide a very nice contrast in flavor, texture, and temperature. A ridged grill pan does a wonderful job. Best of all, the fruits do not have to be peeled!

INGREDIENTS

4 ripe mangoes
3 teaspoons agave nectar, or substitute sugar
Cooking spray
Lime wedges

DIRECTIONS

Heat a grill to high, or heat a grill pan over high heat.

Slice the mangoes. It is always difficult to know exactly where the seeds of mangoes are, so trial and error is the best solution. The goal is to slice the mango into pieces as large as possible that do not include the seed. Place a mango on its side and slice it in half, off center, to miss the seed. Cut the other three sides of the mango in the same way. Next, crosshatch the fruit into squares of about ½ inch. By cutting through the fruit just to the skin but not through it. Make the cuts a half inch apart going one way then do the same the other way to create the crosshatched design.

Prepare the sliced mangoes. Brush a little agave nectar on the cut surfaces of each mango then spray with a little cooking spray. Grill the mangoes, flesh side down, for a minute or 2, or just until they are seared with grill marks, but do not cook them until they are soft and completely heated through. Keeping the firm texture and the contrast between the hot surface and the cooler interior is important. Serve the mangos with the lime wedges.

Quick Fruit Pudding

4 servings

PER SERVING | 140 calories | 2 g protein
35 g carbohydrates | 0 g total fat
(0 g saturated) | 0 mg cholesterol
4 g fiber | 27 g sugar | 75 mg sodium

This creamy dessert is actually a cross between a sorbet and a smoothie. Whatever you call it, it produces a symphony of creamy tropical flavors and is very easy to prepare. It can be made with any soft fruit, such as strawberries or peaches, and it leaves a great deal of room for creativity in terms of ingredients and garnishes, such as mint, nuts, or grated coconut. The only constant is the frozen bananas, which provide both body and flavor. It can be made in a blender or food processor, but I think the processor works best because it is better suited to chopping without added liquid, and it makes it easier to remove all the dessert from the bowl.

INGREDIENTS

2 bananas, peeled, sliced into ½-inch rounds, and frozen on a sheet of aluminum foil

3 cups peeled and chopped mango, or another fruit

2 tablespoons freshly squeezed lime juice

2 teaspoons agave nectar

⅛ teaspoon salt

Mint leaves

DIRECTIONS

Put all the ingredients in the bowl of a food processor fitted with the steel blade or in a blender and process until just liquefied, smooth, and creamy. Garnish with the mint.

Blueberry Frozen Yogurt

About 8 half-cup servings

PER SERVING | 120 calories | 3 g protein
30 g carbohydrates | 0 g total fat
(0 g saturated) | 0 mg cholesterol
1 g fiber | 26 g sugar | 35 mg sodium

This tasty frozen dessert can be made with most fruits, including raspberries, blackberries, and mango. The recipe calls for Splenda instead of sugar, which does leave a slight artificial-sugar aftertaste. But for those who cannot have sugar, it is still a treat. Using part Splenda and part sugar will make it even better, and even when made with all sugar, you still have a low-fat dessert. Because of the small amount of fat and sugar, this freezes very hard, so soften it in a microwave oven before serving. Nutrition calculations are based on ¾ cup sugar and ¼ cup Splenda, which lowers the calories and minimizes the artificial-sugar taste.

INGREDIENTS

2 cups frozen blueberries, not quite thawed

1 cup Splenda or sugar, or a combination

2 cups plain nonfat yogurt

DIRECTIONS

Put all the ingredients for the base into a blender and purée. Pour the base in an ice cream maker and freeze according to the manufacturer's directions. It usually takes between 10 and 20 minutes, depending on how cold the base is.

Grilled Bananas in Coconut Sauce

4 servings

PER SERVING | 170 calories | 1 g protein
39 g carbohydrates | 2 g total fat
(1.5 g saturated) | 0 mg cholesterol
3 g fiber | 23 g sugar | 10 mg sodium

This dessert is perfect to follow a meal of grilled foods. It can be made on an outdoor grill or in a grill pan on the stove.

INGREDIENTS

½ cup lite coconut milk
2 tablespoons agave nectar
1½ teaspoons cornstarch
1 tablespoon water
4 bananas, peeled

DIRECTIONS

Make the coconut sauce. Bring the coconut milk and agave nectar to a simmer in a small saucepan. While it is heating, combine the cornstarch and water. When the liquid begins to simmer, stir in the cornstarch and water and simmer, stirring frequently, until the mixture thickens to sauce consistency.

Grill the bananas and serve. Heat a grill or grill pan on high. Brush the bananas with some of the Coconut Sauce, reserving the remainder, and grill on both sides until they have grill marks and are just beginning to soften. Do not overcook them or they will fall apart. Serve the bananas topped with a little more of the sauce.

Mango Sorbet

8 third-cup servings

PER SERVING | 60 calories | 0 g protein
14 g carbohydrates | 0 g total fat
(0 g saturated) | 0 mg cholesterol
1 g fiber | 13 g sugar | 0 mg sodium

This sorbet has less than 1 teaspoon sugar per serving.

INGREDIENTS

2½ cups peeled, seeded, and chopped mango
3½ tablespoons sugar
Scant ⅔ cup water
½ teaspoon cinnamon, preferably *canela*
½ teaspoon ground allspice
1 tablespoon limoncello

DIRECTIONS

Blend all of the ingredients until puréed. Pour the purée into an ice cream maker and freeze according to the manufacturer's directions. It usually takes between 15 and 20 minutes.

Flan

6 four-ounce servings

PER SERVING | 140 calories
10 g protein | 20 g carbohydrates
2.5 g total fat (1 g saturated)
70 mg cholesterol | 0 g fiber
20 g sugar | 140 mg sodium

This is the best low-fat, low-sugar recipe for Mexico's most famous dessert I have found, and it is very good, especially compared to most of the flans found in Mexican restaurants. It is especially noteworthy when you consider that each serving has only 140 calories and 2.5 grams of fat, compared with a serving of regular flan, which has about 310 calories and 9 grams of fat. To make chocolate flan, simply blend unsweetened cocoa powder into the other ingredients.

INGREDIENTS

1 cup nonfat evaporated milk
1 cup 2% milk
¼ cup nonfat condensed milk
1 teaspoon vanilla extract
2 large eggs
4 egg whites from large eggs
2½ tablespoons unsweetened cocoa powder (optional)
Cooking spray
6 teaspoons agave nectar

DIRECTIONS

Preheat your oven to 325°F.

Make the flan base. Combine the ingredients, except for the cooking spray and agave nectar, in a blender and blend until completely combined, about 1 minute.

Prepare the flan for baking. Spray six 4-ounce oven-safe ramekins with a little cooking spray and place them in a baking dish into which they fit fairly tightly. Fill the ramekins to within ¼-inch of the top with the flan base. Pour enough very hot tap water into the baking dish to come halfway up the sides of the ramekins.

Bake the flan. Put the baking dish with the filled ramekins in the oven for 40 minutes, or until the flans are set and just firm. Remove the baking dish from the oven and the ramekins from the dish. Allow the flans to cool, then cover them with plastic wrap and refrigerate until cold. Serve each flan topped with 1 teaspoon agave nectar.

Bibliography

Andrews, Jean. *Peppers: The Domesticated Capsicums*. University of Texas Press, 1984.

Bayless, Rick, with Deann Groen Bayless. *Authentic Mexican: Regional Cooking from the Heart of Mexico*. William Morrow, 1987.

Bays, Jan Chozen, M.D. "Mindful Eating: The French Paradox." *Psychology Today* (March 2009).

Caraza Campos, Laura B. de. *La cocina de Laura*. Promexa, 1997.

Cardona, Gloria. *Delicias vegetarianas de México*. Editorial Pax, 2006.

Clark, Melissa. "Once a Villain: Coconut Oil Charms the Health Food World." *New York Times* (March 1, 2011).

Curtis, Susan. *The Santa Fe School of Cooking Cookbook*. Gibbs-Smith, 1995.

De'Angeli, Alicia Gironella, and Jorge De'Angeli. *Gran libro de la cocina mexicana*. Larousse, 1988.

Delgado, Ana Laura, and María Stoopen. *La cocina veracruzana*. Gobierno del Estado de Veracruz, 1992.

Flores, Carlotta. *El Charro Café: The Tastes and Traditions of Tucson*. Fisher Books, 1998.

Fraser, Laura. "The French Paradox." Salon.com, February 4, 2000.

Gilliland, Tom, and Miguel Ravago. *Fonda San Miguel: Thirty Years of Food and Art*. Shearer Publishing, 2005.

Griggs, Josephine C. *A Family Affair*. J. C. Griggs and E. N. Smith-Bronson Printing, 1968.

Katz, S. H., et al. "Traditional Maize Processing Techniques in the New World." *Science* (May 1974).

Kennedy, Diana. *The Cuisines of Mexico*. Harper & Row, 1972.

———. *My Mexico*. Clarkson Potter, 1998.

———. *Recipes from the Regional Cooks of Mexico*. Harper & Row, 1978.

Martínez, Zarela, with Anne Mendelson. *Zarela's Veracruz*. Houghton Mifflin, 2001.

McMahan, Jacqueline Higuera. *The Salsa Book*. Olive Press, 1986.

Miller, Mark. *Tacos*. Ten Speed Press, 2009.

———, Stephan Pyles, and John Sedlar. *Tamales*. Macmillan, 1997.

Molinar, Rita. *Dulces mexicanos*. Editorial Pax, 1991.

Muñoz Zurita, Ricardo. *Verde en la cocina mexicana*. Fundación Herdez, 1999.

Nigh, Kippy. *México a mi sazón*. Panorama Editorial, 1999.

Peyton, James W. *El Norte: The Cuisine of Northern Mexico*. Red Crane Books, 1990.

———. *La Cocina de la Frontera: Mexican-American Cooking from the Southwest*. Red Crane Books, 1994.

———. *Jim Peyton's New Cooking from Old Mexico*. Red Crane Books, 1999.

———. *Jim Peyton's The Very Best of Tex-Mex Cooking, plus Texas Barbecue and Texas Chile*. Maverick Publishing, 2005.

Quintana, Patricia. *Cuisine of the Water Gods*. Simon & Schuster, 1994.

Sacks, Frank M., et al. "Comparison of Weight-Loss Diets with Different Compositions of Fat, Protein, and Carbohydrates." *New England Journal of Medicine* (February 26, 2009).

Shulman, Martha Rose. *Mexican Light: Exciting, Healthy Dishes from the Border and Beyond*. Bantam Books, 1996.

Telcholz, Nina. "What If Bad Fat Is Actually Good for You?" *Men's Health* (May 7, 2009).

Urdaneta, María Luisa, and Daryl F. Kanter. *Deleites de la Cocina Mexicana: A Bilingual Cookbook*. University of Texas Press, 1996.

Ventura, Emily, et al. "Reduction in Risk Factors for Type 2 Diabetes Mellitus in Response to a Low-Sugar, High-Fiber Dietary Intervention in Overweight Latino Adolescents." *JAMA Pediatrics* (April 2009).

Von Bremzen, Anya. *The New Spanish Table*. New York: Workman, 2005.

Zamudio, María Luisa, and Alida Gutiérrez Zamora. *Las recetas de mi mamá: Cocina jarocha*. Litográfica Turmex.

Recipe Index

General Index